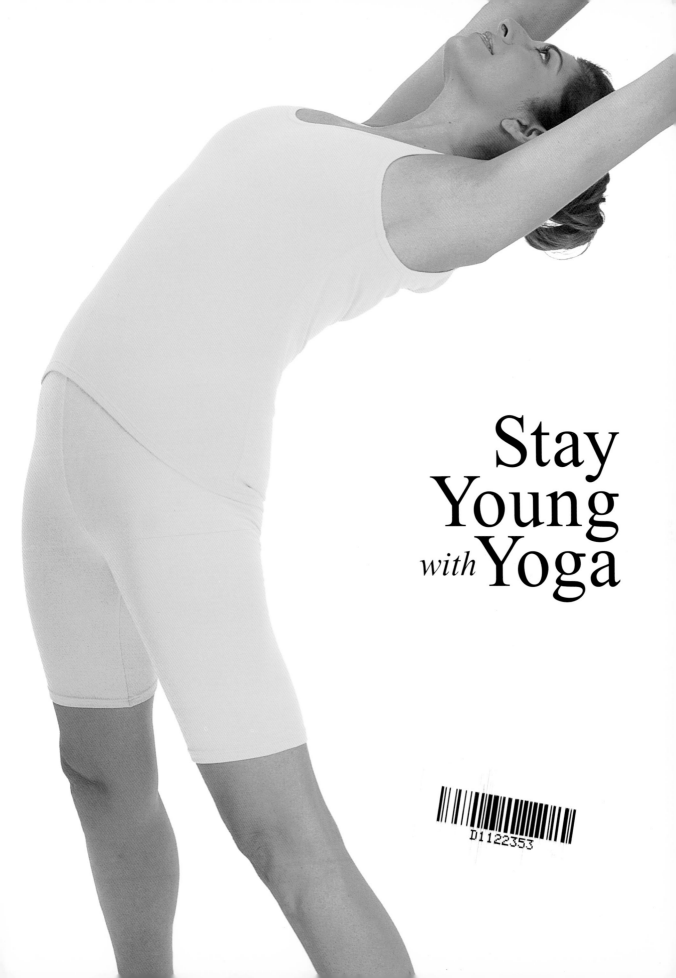

Stay
Young
with Yoga

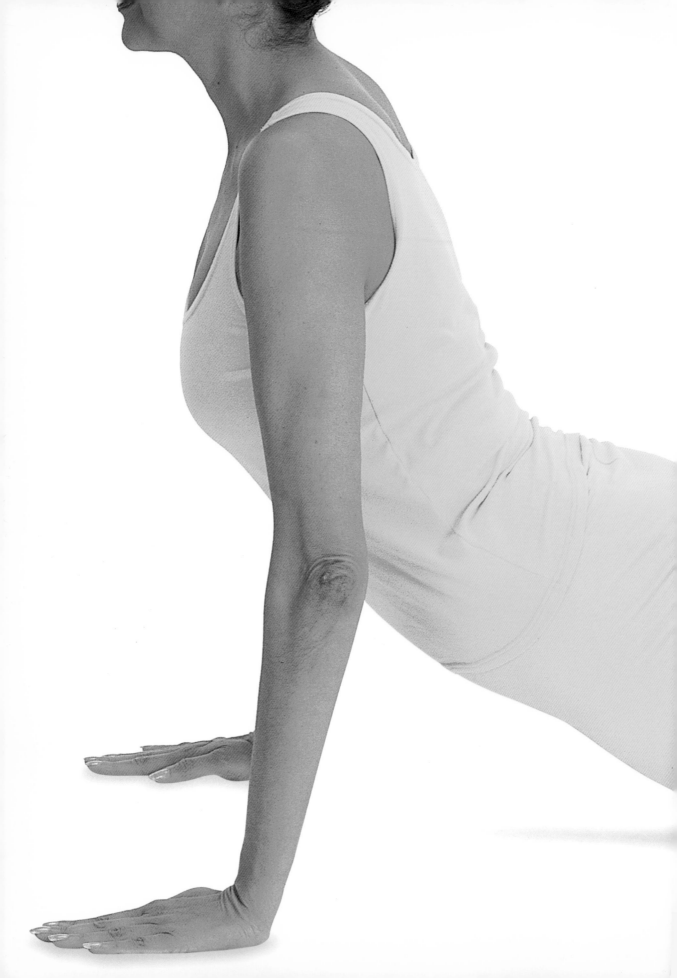

Stay Young *with* Yoga

Vimla Lalvani

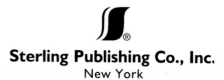

Sterling Publishing Co., Inc.
New York

Library of Congress
Cataloging-in-Publication Data Available

10 9 8 7 6 5 4 3 2 1

Published in 2001 by Sterling Publishing Company, Inc
387 Park Avenue South, New York, N.Y. 10016

First published in Great Britain in 1998 under the title
Stop the Age Clock by Hamlyn, an imprint of
Octopus Publishing Group Limited, 2–4 Heron Quays, London, E14 4JP
© The Natural Therapy Company Limited, 1998
Design © Octopus Publishing Group Limited, 1998
Photographs © Octopus Publishing Group Limited, 1998

Distributed in Canada by Sterling Publishing
c/o Canadian Manda Group, One Atlantic Avenue, Suite 105
Toronto, Ontario, Canada M6K 3E7

Printed and bound in China

Sterling ISBN 0-8069-5890-1

Safety Note
It is advisable to check with your doctor before embarking on any
exercise program. Yoga should not be considered a replacement for
professional medical treatment; a physician should be consulted in all
matters relating to health and particularly in respect of pregnancy and
any symptoms which may require diagnosis or medical attention. While
the advice and information in this book is believed to be accurate and
the step-by-step instructions have been devised to avoid strain, neither
the author nor the publisher can accept any legal responsibility for any
injury sustained while following the exercises.

CONTENTS

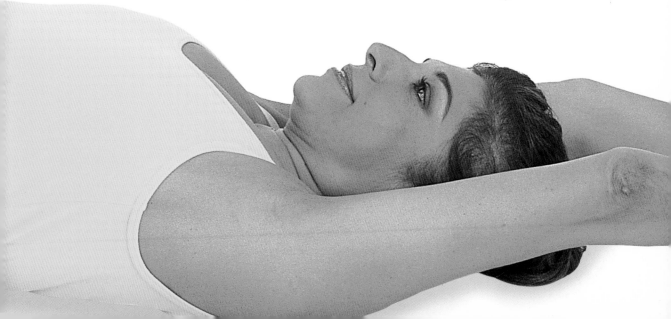

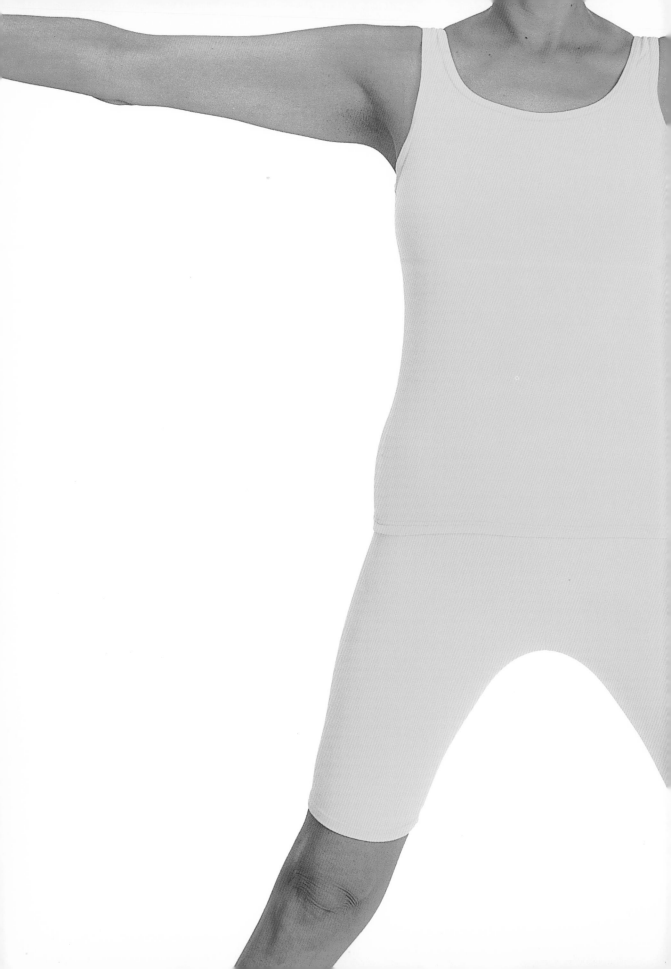

INTRODUCTION

The quest for eternal youth is universal and never-ending. Even the earliest records of human civilizations provide evidence of elixirs and potions used to preserve youth and beauty, while numerous scientists today are engaged in a search for new techniques with which to hold the ageing process at bay. Millions of pounds are spent by the public each year on anti-ageing creams and body treatments and some people resort to cosmetic surgery to restore the appearance of youth.

Much of this effort is futile, however. Creams cannot perform miracles and cosmetic surgery merely provides a temporary reprieve that usually leads to further and more drastic encounters with the surgeon's scalpel. But, even though we cannot reverse the ageing process altogether, we *can* learn to outwit the process so we can stay young and full of energy for a greater length of time.

To most people, the word 'youthful' conjures up someone with boundless energy and an inquisitive mind, a person with a beautifully toned and flexible body, sparkling eyes and a glowing complexion – and I have designed a new system of movement that will help you match this description whatever your age. It will counteract the effects of time by regulating your metabolism, balancing your hormonal system, raising your energy levels, focusing your mind and keeping your spine supple. This technique is based on the ancient system of yoga combined with movement so the body flows in smooth, graceful motion. As the spine becomes more flexible energy flows more freely throughout the system, increasing vitality, while correct yoga breathing rejuvenates the entire mind and body.

There is a proverb in yoga philosophy that says the day you begin your yoga practice the age clock stops. Yoga exercises also regulate the metabolism so there is no weight gain or loss. Many men and women complain about middle-aged spread but do not realize that because their metabolism has slowed down they have to burn more calories through exercise or decrease their calorie intake in their diets. Once you reach balance through yoga exercises, however, you will not need to diet to maintain your weight.

The ageing body

The first signs of ageing are physical, with skin and muscle beginning to sag. We refer to this slackened muscle as flab and ridding ourselves of it is considered a prerequisite to maintaining a youthful, attractive appearance. The intense stretching of the muscles that takes place in yoga will not only tighten and tone each muscle group but will also eliminate the fat cells around each muscle. The result will be a tight and firm body with no excess flab.

As people age they also tend to feel lethargic and totally lacking in energy. Most people lead sedentary lives and never quite make the commitment to improving their physical health until something goes wrong. This can be a

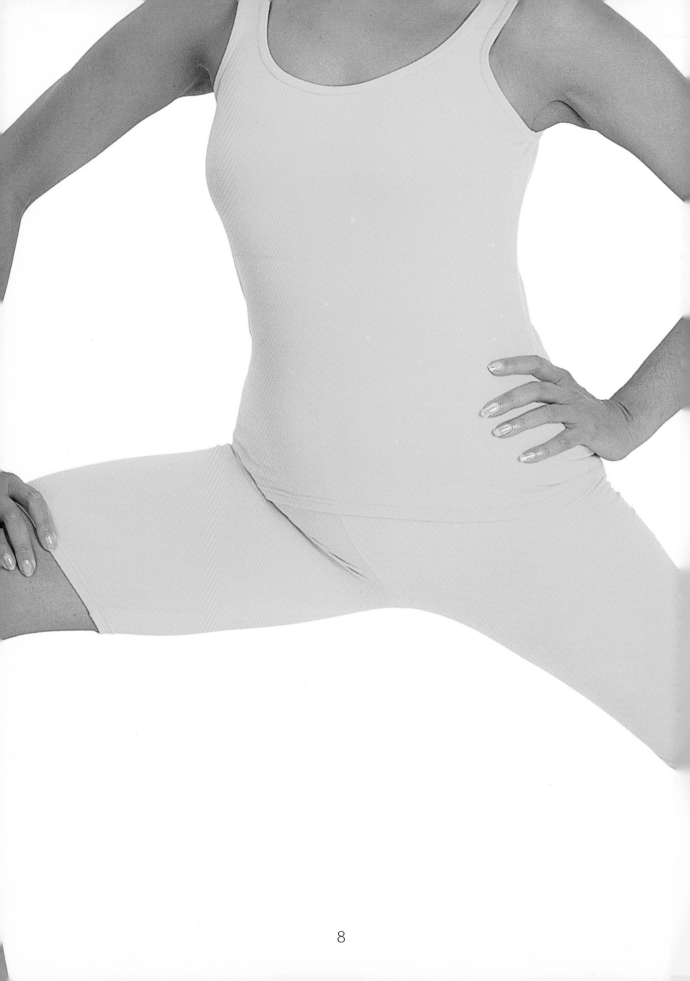

dangerous attitude; it is far more important to take preventive measures than to take good health for granted and then try to find a cure after illness has struck. When a car breaks down due to lack of maintenance we can buy a new one to replace the old, but as we have only one body we must never give it a chance to decay. This is where yoga philosophy comes in, for it is a well-developed science that maintains the body to its highest standard.

The yoga poses require you to twist and turn in every direction. This activity stimulates the nerves and carries fresh blood to each organ in the body. When it is combined with correct breathing each organ receives a fresh supply of pure oxygen. Holding the pose helps to alter the energy in the system, giving it a boost of vitality.

The ageing mind

Many people fear the prospect of growing old and see it as inevitably a negative experience. However, the saying that you are as old as you look and feel has a lot of truth in it. If you feel old you will look dramatically different from a person with a youthful attitude. I'm sure we all know people who seem to have been born old: their bodies are stiff and they seem to lack a sense of joy and spontaneity. A person who has excellent health and enjoys daily living is much more attractive at any age than a dull person who complains constantly about getting old. The secret

of staying young is to have an agile and curious mind that is constantly fascinated by new thoughts and trends. At the age of 100, my grandfather would see a film every Saturday afternoon whatever the subject matter. It was his way of staying in touch with the constantly changing world and keeping his mind alert.

It is important to feed brain cells with a fresh blood supply to combat senility and memory loss, and in yoga we perform postures where the legs are positioned over the head to allow the blood to rush to the brain to soothe the nervous system. Simply dropping the head forward when you are standing upright has the same effect.

Degenerative diseases

Many people believe that degenerative diseases such as arthritis, osteoporosis and urinary and digestive disorders are synonymous with growing old. This is a myth, for we can prolong good health by learning to be in tune with our bodies. We must consider what we eat and drink and understand why it is necessary not to overload the body with unwanted toxins. Food is fuel for the entire system, so each of us must eat correctly according to our personal needs. In most cases when the immune system is strong the physical body will fight against any illness, even if it is of genetic origin. Yoga exercises boost the entire immune system to help prevent ill health from occurring in any age group. If ailments do occur, yoga can help to alleviate the symptoms and in some cases can eliminate the condition completely

Ayurveda

Ayurvedic medicine comes from the same ancient century of wisdom and intellect as the *Yoga Sutras*. Ayurveda means 'the science of life', and according to its philosophy good physical health includes mental, physical and spiritual integration. Even though each case is treated as individual, people are considered to fall into three categories that relate to the elements of air, fire, and water. These forces are associated with temperament, physical attributes and liking for particular foods as well as natural resistance or weaknesses to certain diseases. Most people are a combination of two categories.

The Vata or air person is tall, thin and wiry, impatient, restless and talkative. These people love salty, spicy and savory foods and are prone to colds and flu, diseases of the nervous system, arthritis and mental disorders. Their immune system is weak and variable and their resistance to disease is poor.

The Pitta or fire person is moderate in height and physique, hates the heat and is constantly hungry and thirsty. Pitta people are very active and are irritable and easily angered. They are determined, passionate, and love conflict. Their resistance to disease is moderate and they are prone to infections and inflammatory diseases.

Those with Kapha or water constitution are short, stout and have a well-developed physique. They like to exercise but are slower in speech and action than Vata and Pitta people. They love sweet, rich foods and wines. They are resistant to disease and have a strong immune system, but they are prone to respiratory problems and produce mucus in the lungs and sinus passages.

When environmental conditions are stable good health among all types seems to be regulated, but when stressful conditions or major changes occur illnesses can affect the mental and physical harmony of the individual. Such illness can be avoided by taking action to prolong good health and increase longevity.

Breathing correctly

In yoga philosophy, breathing is the essence of each movement. Every exercise begins with a deep inhalation and this breath is directed into the bloodstream. The way you breath has a direct effect on how young you look. A shallow breath does not have a chance to circulate through the internal organs as well as an intense breath, which directly enters each cell and rejuvenates it.

Most people breathe from the chest and raise their shoulders simultaneously so the breath is restricted. In fact, the correct action is in the lower abdomen only so that the lungs are able to fill to their full capacity. During the yoga exercises the breath moves into the specific organ that is being stimulated. There is a tendency to open the mouth when the position becomes difficult to hold but this is the moment to deepen the breath to increase oxygen throughout the system; opening the mouth will allow valuable oxygen to escape.

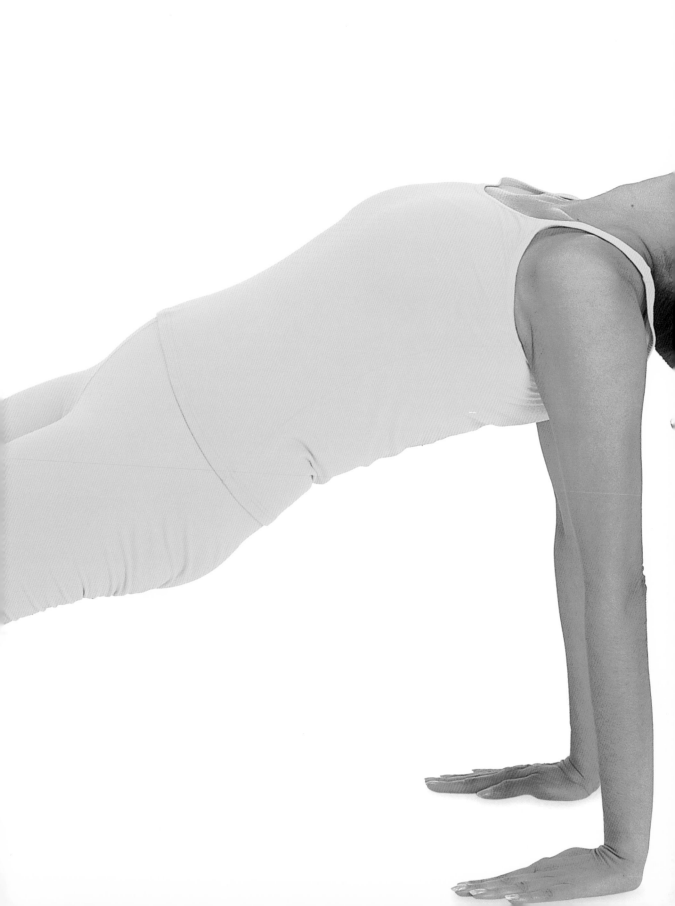

HOW TO USE THIS BOOK

Even though I have divided the exercises in this book into a workout for each of 10 days they can be continued indefinitely to tone and strengthen the body and correct certain conditions and ailments. I have focused on the most important mental and physical aspects that plague many people and have designed an exercise regime for each problem area. These sections can be combined, depending on how much time you have, or you can choose the exercise plan according to your specific needs. The step-by-step text within the 10 day plan corresponds to the sequence of images which run along the top of each page in this section.

Always begin with the Warm-up to avoid any strain or injury and to prepare your body for the exercise plan that you select. The Round-the-Body routine is a top-to-toe fitness program that targets specific areas of the body and there are also remedial exercises for particular areas of concern. They can be practised on their own or combined with any of the other routines.

Safety guidelines

There are important guidelines that must be followed in order to ensure that you gain all the benefits of yoga to the full and that you do not injure or strain yourself while adopting any of the poses in this book.

• These exercises are designed for people in a normal state of health. As is the case with any fitness program, if you feel unfit or unwell or are recovering from any injury, or if you are pregnant, have high blood pressure or suffer from any medical disorder, you must consult your doctor before you embark upon any of the exercises.

• It is important to follow the instructions in the exercises and to read through each exercise before beginning it.

• Never rush the movements. Do not jerk your body and stop immediately if you experience any sharp pain or strain. Never try to push yourself and always do the pose only to your own capability.

• Pay particular attention to your breathing in order to help relax and focus your mind. Let your deep breathing also relax your body and allow the stretched muscles and ligaments to carry more energy to the muscle fibers. Pay attention to your posture, too, and make sure that you always stand, sit or kneel upright.

• When you are in a standing pose you will often be required to balance upon one leg. Keep this leg straight by lifting the muscle above the kneecap. Be careful not to hyperextend or lock the knee as this can cause injury.

• Choose a warm, quiet, well-ventilated place in which to embark upon any yoga exercises.

• Exercise barefoot so that you can grip the floor with your toes. Make sure you exercise on an even, non-slip surface. You may find it more comfortable to use a mat for the floor exercises.

• Do not attempt yoga exercises on a full stomach – allow an interval of one hour after a light meal and four hours after a heavy meal.

• Always follow the recommended warm-up before attempting the exercises. You can loosen your muscles even more by taking a shower first.

• Remember these basic principles: mental and spiritual control of movements; physical awareness of postures and movements; slow and deliberate movements; relaxation during movements; go only as far as is comfortable.

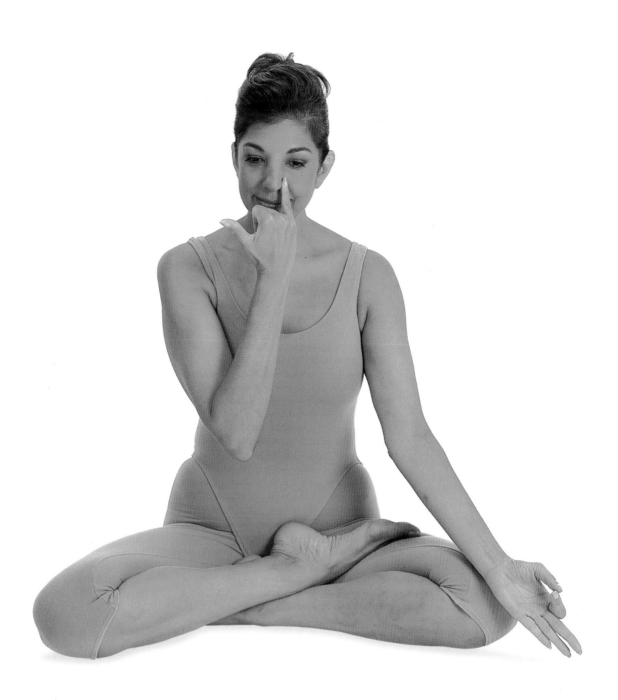

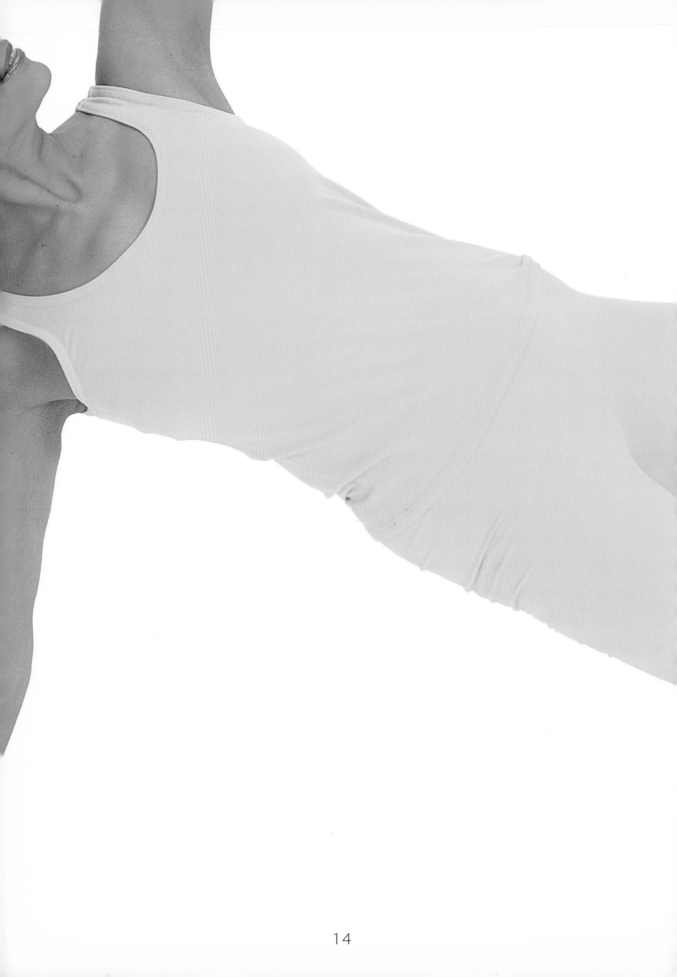

EXERCISES

I have designed ten exercise routines with different objectives, each taking about ten minutes to do. Day One reduces tension in the muscle groups; Day Two improves the circulation to prevent stiffness in the joints; Day Three tones the parts of the body that show the first signs of ageing; Day Four strengthens the lower back to alleviate back pain; Day Five opens the chest area to unblock trapped energy in the spine; Day Six works on the hip joints to increase blood flow to the lower body; Day Seven energizes the entire system; Day Eight concentrates and focuses the mind; Day Nine teaches correct breathing to rejuvenate the system; and Day Ten calms the nervous system to restore harmony to mind and body.

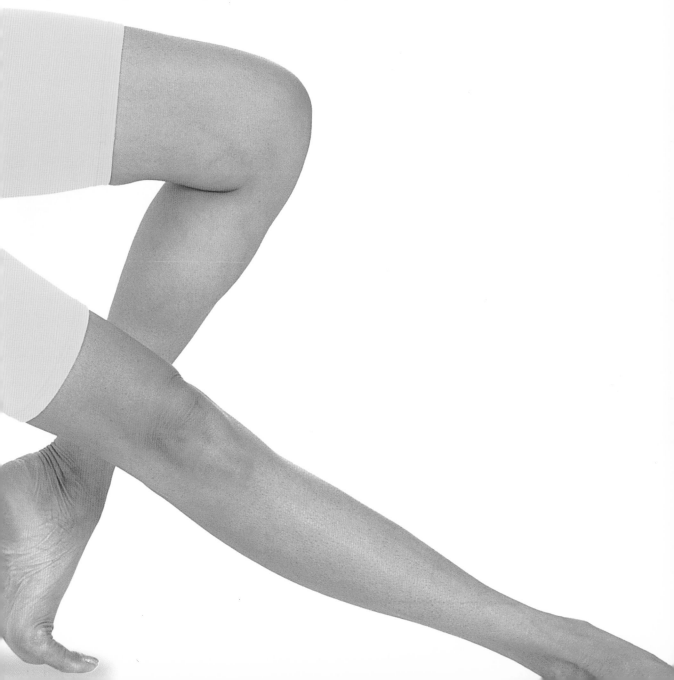

WARM-UP

It is always very important to warm up the body first before you begin any exercise regime. These exercises will slowly allow the energy to flow through the muscle groups so you can easily stretch without causing any strain or injury to the body. Always concentrate on the breathing pattern so that the movements will be slow and graceful. Before you begin any exercise, stand tall with your feet together and imagine there is a string pulling you upwards from the top of your head; this is known as 'perfect posture'. Inhale and exhale at least five times to restore inner calm and focus your attention on yourself. Concentrate upon the action you are about to perform.

Place your feet on the floor and distribute your weight evenly between your toes and heels. Every muscle in your entire body should be working as you lift upwards. Tighten your tummy and buttock muscles and tuck your tailbone under so your spine is in perfect alignment. Open your shoulder blades, drop them downwards and keep your chin level. Begin by breathing deeply from the diaphragm through the nose. Inhale and exhale deeply for 5–7 seconds. ▶ Inhale and rise up on to your toes, keeping yourself in perfect balance and breathing normally while you are holding the pose. Hold for 3 seconds. ▶ Exhale and lower your heels down to the floor. Repeat. ▶

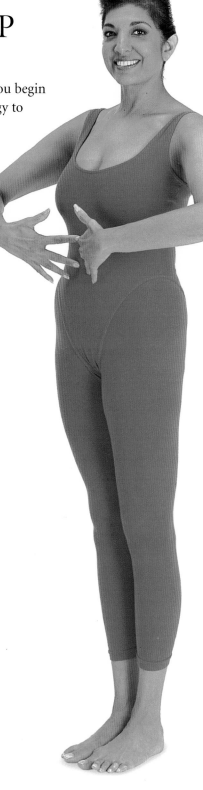

1

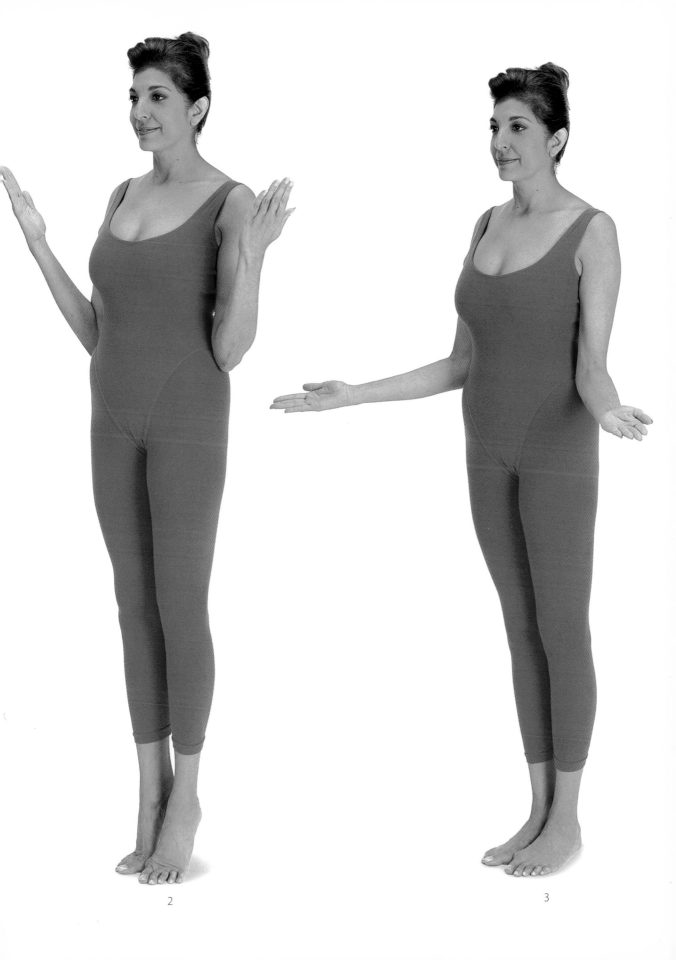

2

3

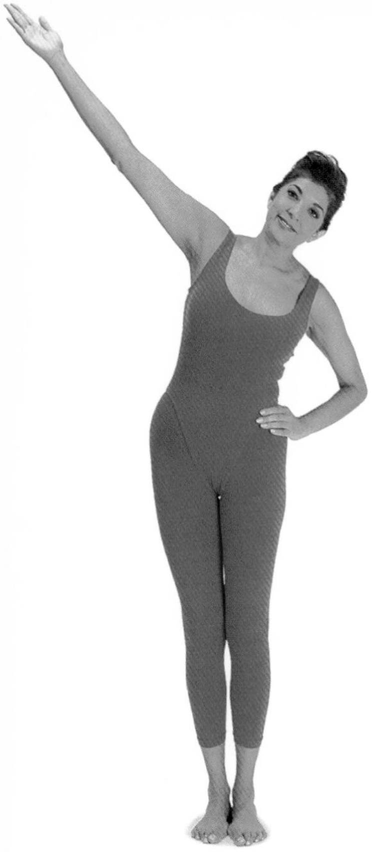

Take your left hand to your waist. Inhale, and sweep your right arm up from your right side.
▶Take your right arm over your head as you stretch your upper body from the waist as far as you can to the left. Keep both hips square. Hold for at least 5 seconds, breathing deeply and evenly.
▶Take your right hand to your waist and extend your left arm in a diagonal line to the shoulder.
▶ Inhale and take your arm over your head, stretching from the waist in a circular motion. Exhale and breathe normally for 5–7 seconds.

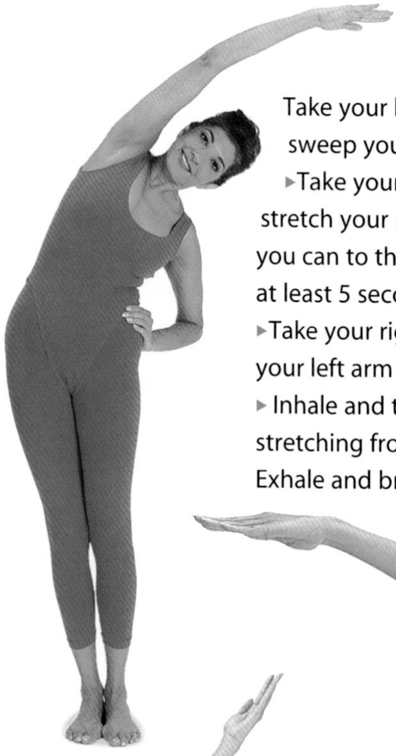

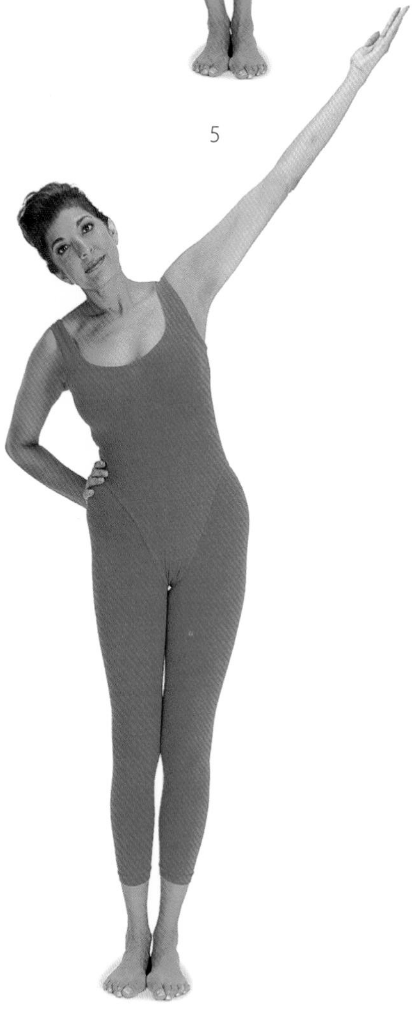

4

5

6

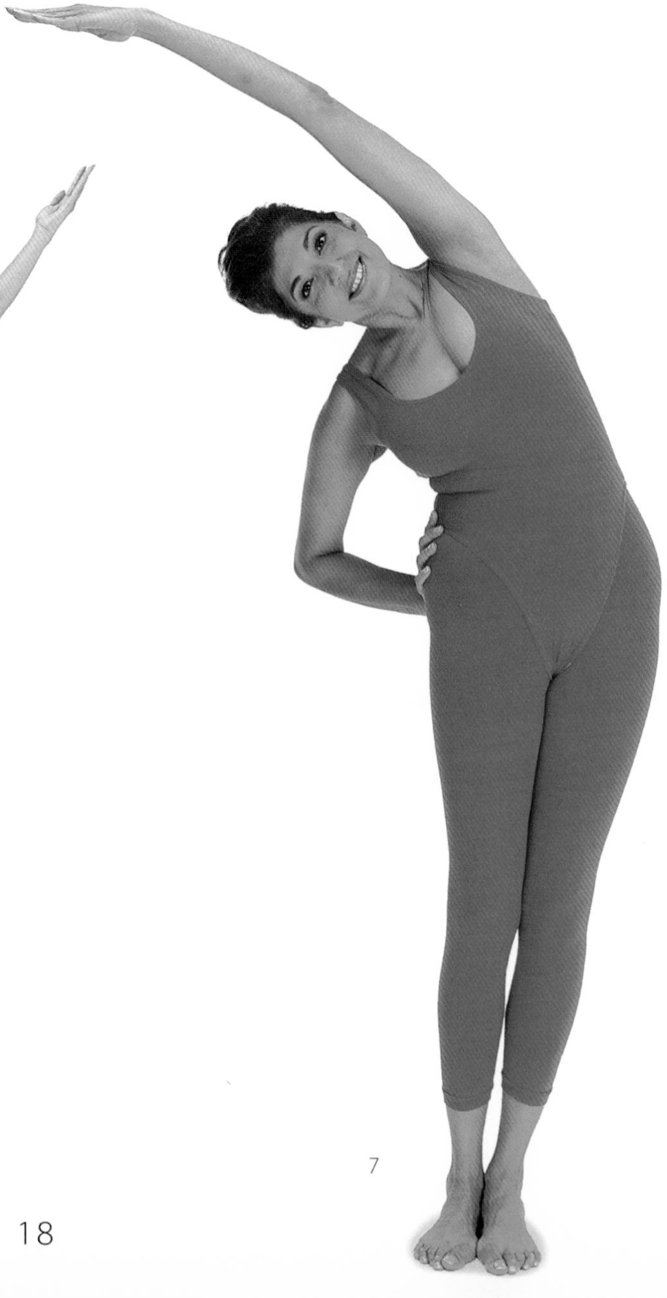

7

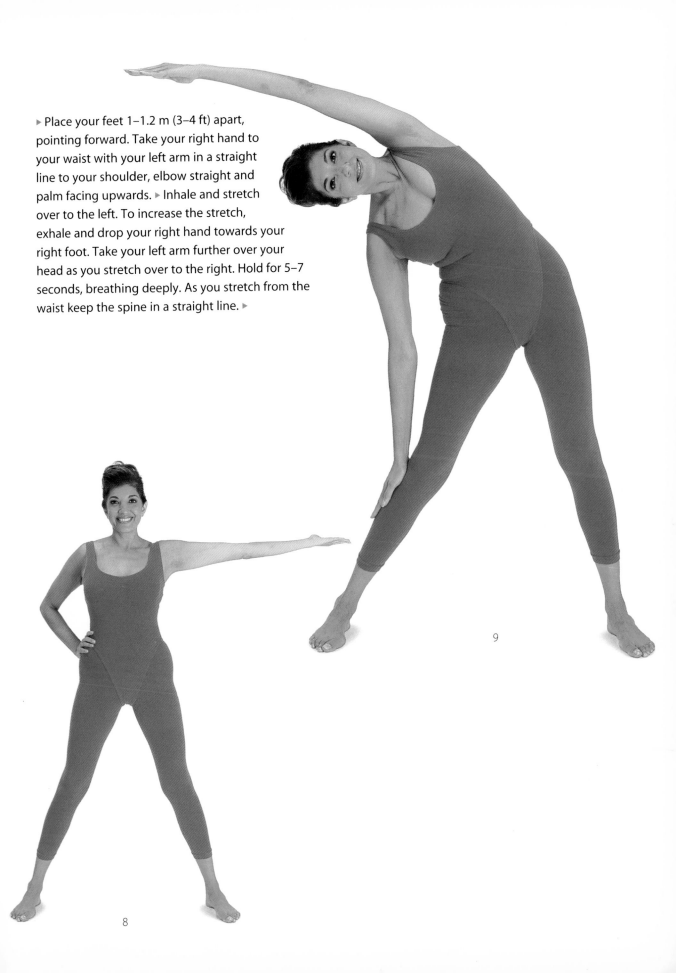

▸ Place your feet 1–1.2 m (3–4 ft) apart, pointing forward. Take your right hand to your waist with your left arm in a straight line to your shoulder, elbow straight and palm facing upwards. ▸ Inhale and stretch over to the left. To increase the stretch, exhale and drop your right hand towards your right foot. Take your left arm further over your head as you stretch over to the right. Hold for 5–7 seconds, breathing deeply. As you stretch from the waist keep the spine in a straight line. ▸

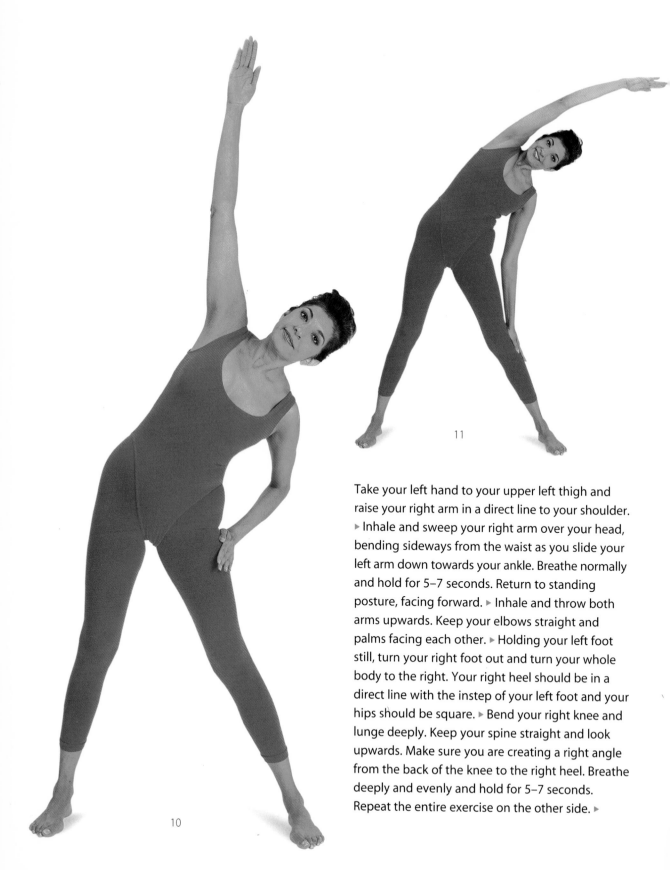

10

11

Take your left hand to your upper left thigh and raise your right arm in a direct line to your shoulder. ▸ Inhale and sweep your right arm over your head, bending sideways from the waist as you slide your left arm down towards your ankle. Breathe normally and hold for 5–7 seconds. Return to standing posture, facing forward. ▸ Inhale and throw both arms upwards. Keep your elbows straight and palms facing each other. ▸ Holding your left foot still, turn your right foot out and turn your whole body to the right. Your right heel should be in a direct line with the instep of your left foot and your hips should be square. ▸ Bend your right knee and lunge deeply. Keep your spine straight and look upwards. Make sure you are creating a right angle from the back of the knee to the right heel. Breathe deeply and evenly and hold for 5–7 seconds. Repeat the entire exercise on the other side. ▸

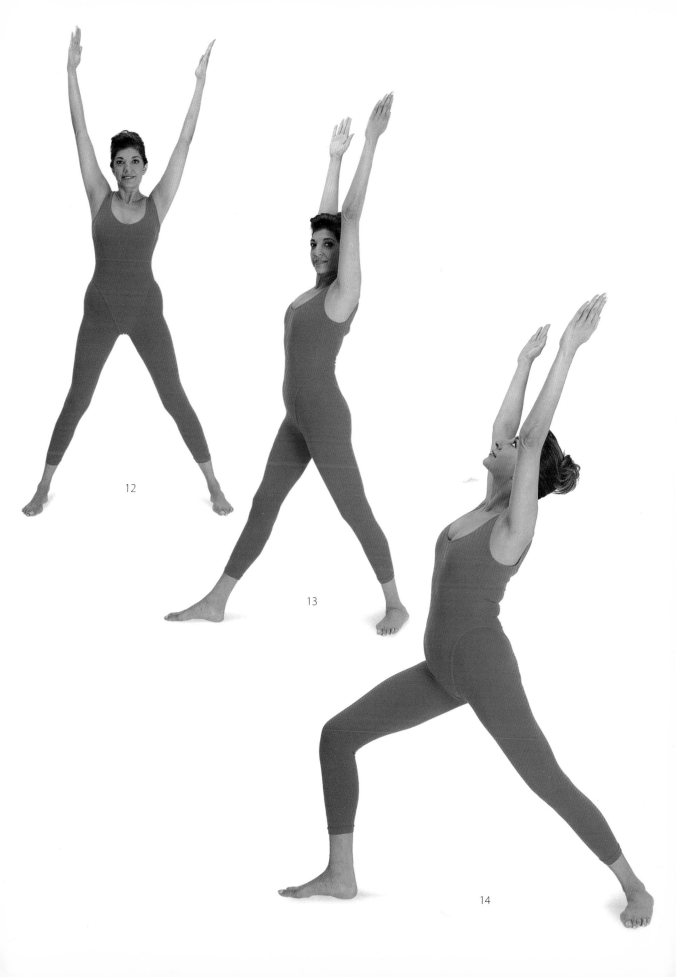

12

13

14

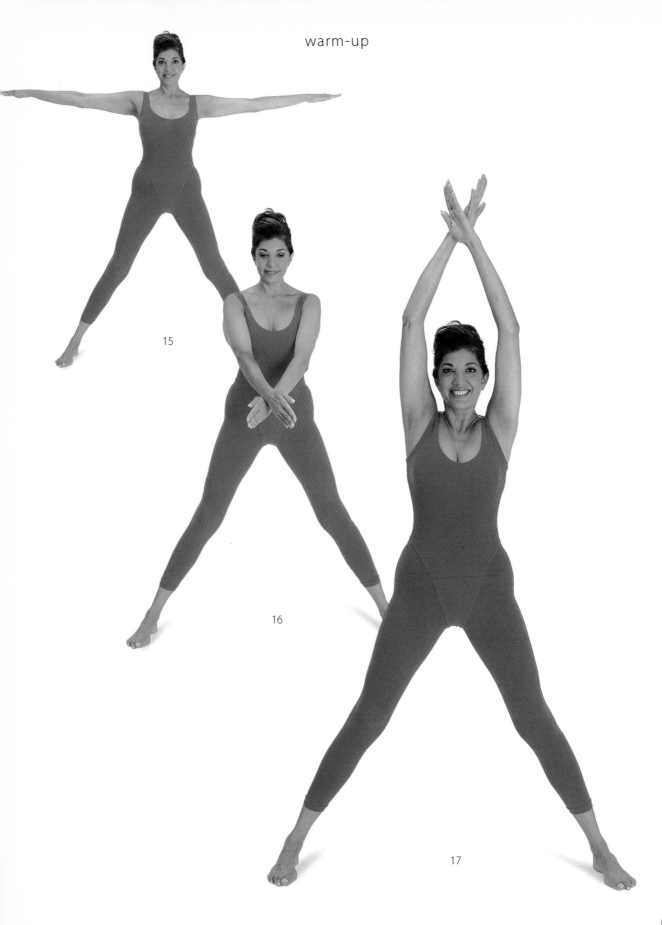

15

16

17

Straighten your leg and turn your body to face forward. Take your arms down to the side, keeping your elbows straight and fingertips together. Make sure your feet still face forward and your knees are straight. ▶ Inhale and take your arms down in front of you, crossing your wrists. Focus your attention on your hands. ▶ Exhale and take your arms up in front of your face, raising them over your head. ▶ Inhale and as you exhale release both hands with a burst of energy. Leaving your arms up, inhale and as you exhale drop your body forward, taking your arms down to the floor. ▶ Breathe deeply and evenly and allow your natural body weight to take you down further. If your spine is stiff and you are unable to lower yourself to the floor do not force or jerk your body. You will be surprised at how fast your suppleness and flexibility will improve with this simple exercise. Hold for 5–7 seconds. ▶ Pull your tummy muscles up and stretch further, holding your ankles and lowering your head towards the floor. Hold for 5 seconds then slowly uncurl the spine and return to standing position.

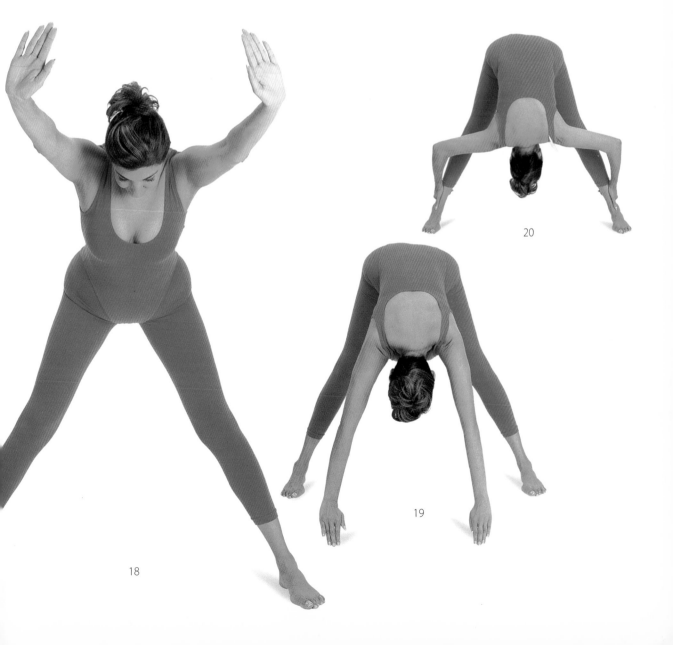

18

19

20

Day one
STRESS

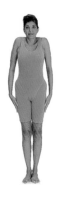 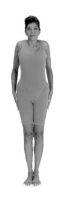

In today's hectic world it is impossible to avoid stress, but we can learn to cope with it. Yoga provides the natural solution as it not only releases the tension in the muscle groups through intense stretching but also, through deep breathing techniques, calms and soothes the brain and relaxes the entire nervous system. In this section we will be concentrating on the areas such as the neck and shoulders which hold tension and on releasing the stress trapped in the internal organs. When people are stressed, weak organs are depleted of energy and the healthy organs become overworked as they try to compensate. This produces an imbalance in the body and, wherever there is a weak spot, a symptom will occur – which is why people suffering from stress can experience a range of different symptoms.

Stand with your feet together in perfect posture. Think of all the tension trapped in your neck and shoulders. Inhale and lift your shoulders towards your ears as high as possible. ▶ Exhale and drop your shoulders. Repeat the exercise at least twice until you feel your shoulders loosen up. ▶ Inhale and roll your shoulders forwards and upwards, and exhale as you take them backwards and down in a circle. Repeat twice in the same direction. Focus on your breathing and as you exhale feel all the tension leaving the body. ▶ Drop your chin down into the chest, inhale, and begin slowly to roll your head around in a circle to the right. It is very important to keep your shoulders even and roll only your head. ▶ Drop your head to the back, exhale and continue to take your head around to the starting position. If you feel any extra stiffness in a particular area, stop and breathe through the tension until you feel comfortable in the position. Repeat the entire head roll to the right side and then repeat the entire exercise twice to the left. ▶

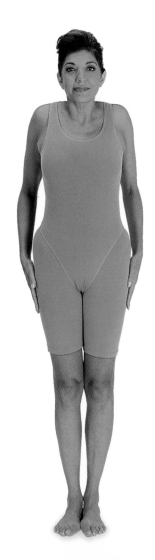

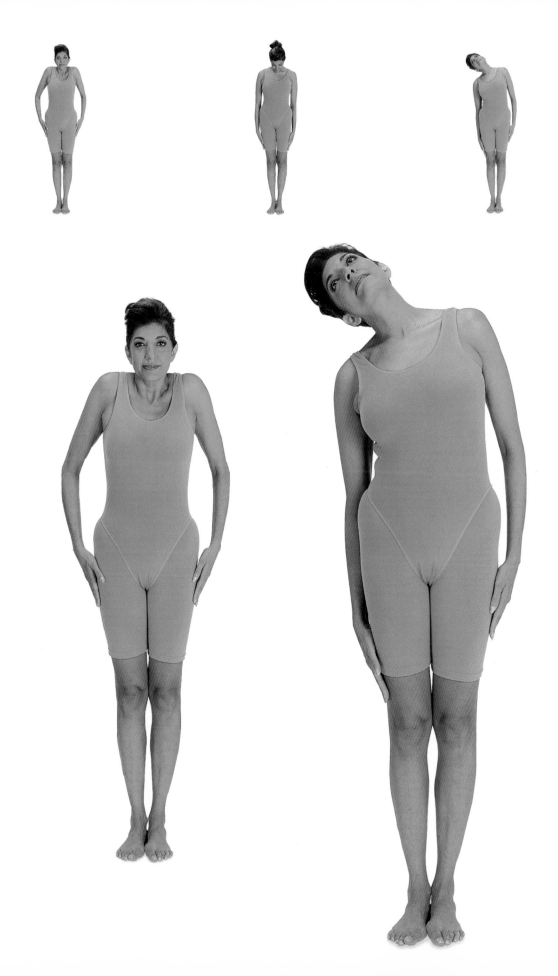

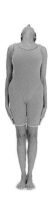 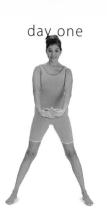

day one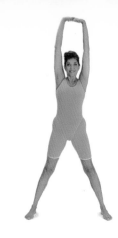

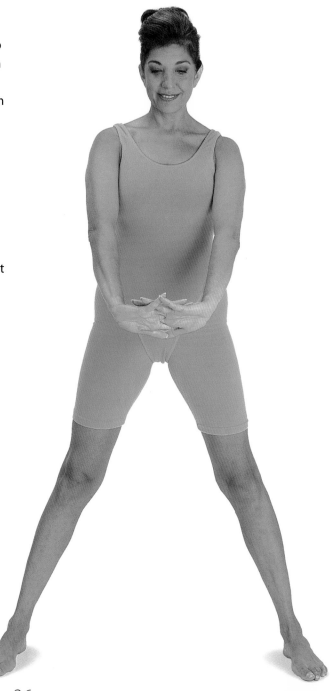

Inhale and drop your head back. Exhale, and drop your chin forward. Repeat. Backache is a common symptom of stress; this next exercise releases tension in the entire spine. ▸ Take your feet 1–1.2 m (3–4 ft) apart, toes pointing forward. Lift the muscle above each kneecap to help you with balance and stand erect. Clasp your fingertips in front of you and look downwards towards your hands. ▸ Inhale and take your arms forward in a circle over your head. Keep your eyes focused on your fingertips. Exhale and look forward. ▸ Inhale and take both arms to the left. ▸ Exhale and turn your body forward to the floor. It is very important to keep the spine straight. ▸ Reaching from the tailbone, sweep your arms in a wide circular movement so your arms reach forward and your palms touch the floor. If you are unable to reach the floor, bend your knees to ease the stretch. ▸

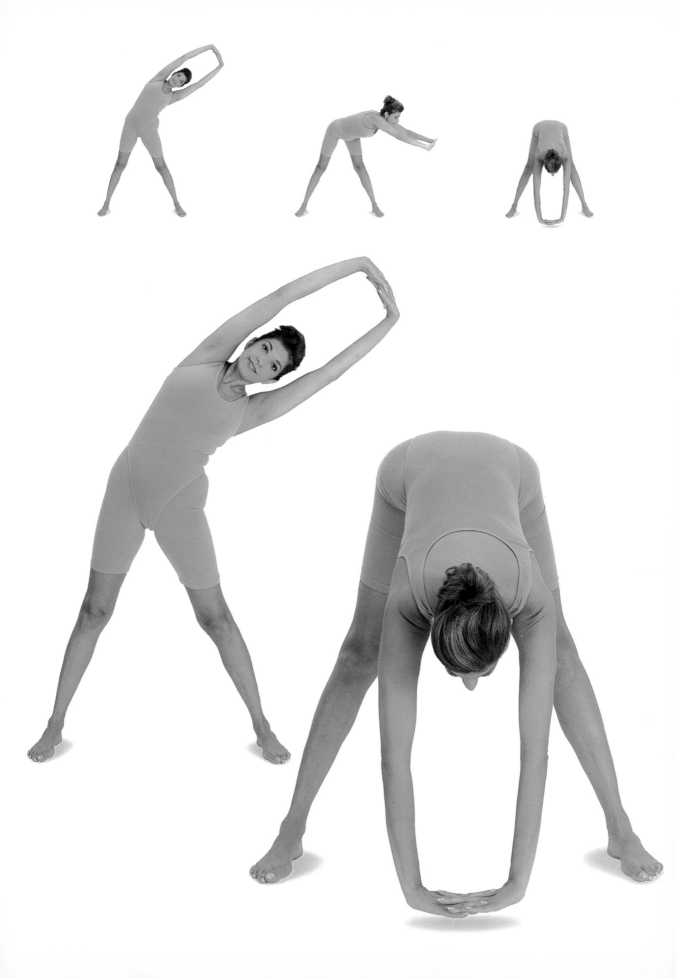

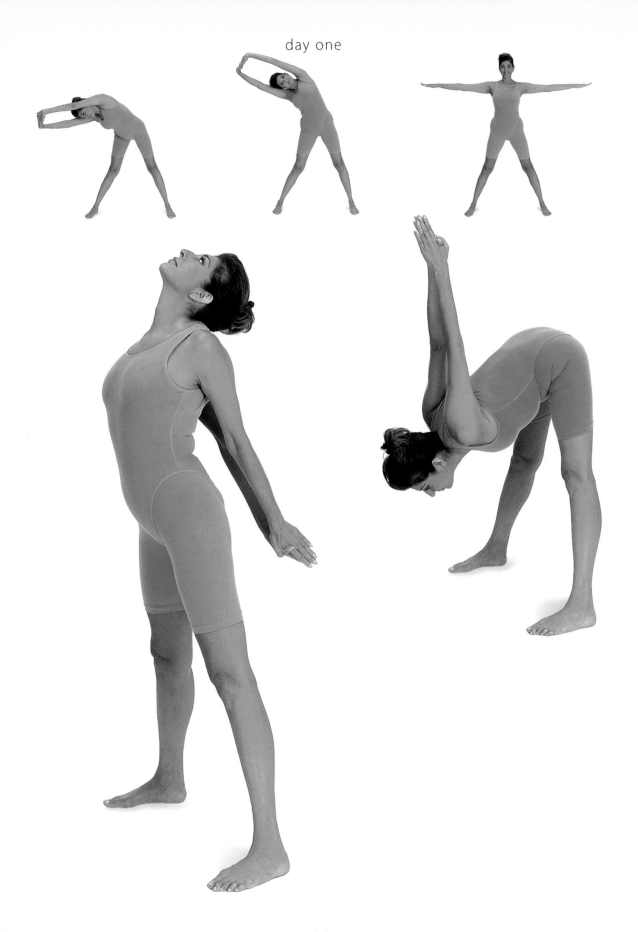

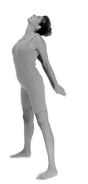
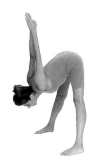
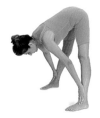

Still clasping your hands together, continue to take your arms round to the right, looking down towards the floor. ▶ Straighten the spine from the tailbone and look forward, keeping the top of the head in line with the fingertips. ▶ Return to standing position and as you exhale release your arms so both are in a straight line to your shoulders. ▶ Take your arms behind your back. Cross your thumbs and place your palms together, keeping your fingertips together. Straighten your elbows and push your shoulders down. ▶ Looking upwards, inhale and as you continue to stretch the neck and chin, exhale and slowly stretch forward from the tailbone, keeping the spine straight. Breathe deeply and evenly and hold for 5–7 seconds. As you breathe, try to keep your elbows straight and lift your arms up as high as possible. This releases all the tension in the upper back, neck, and shoulders. ▶ Keeping your spine straight, release your arms and place your hands on your ankles. ▶

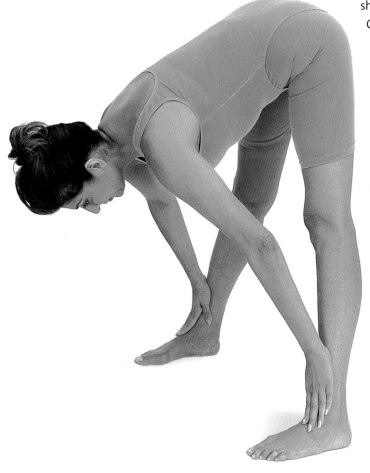

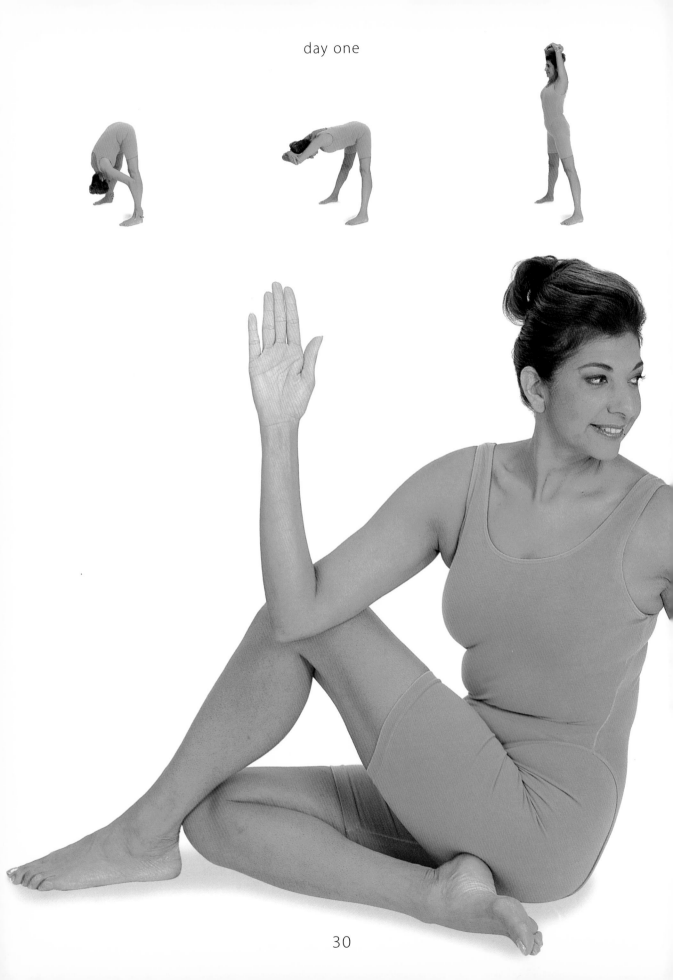

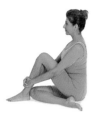 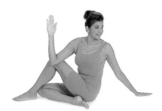 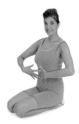

Inhale and as you exhale, bend the elbows, curve the spine and draw your forehead down between your legs. Breathe deeply and hold for 5 seconds. ▶ Fold your arms over your head, holding onto your elbows. Inhale, pull your tummy muscles in and straighten your spine so your head is in line with your tailbone. Exhale and hold the position for 5 seconds. ▶ On the inhalation, return to standing position, keeping your arms overhead. ▶ Now sit on the floor and bend your right leg so your knee is in a direct line to your right hipbone. Place your left foot directly in front of the right knee so the heel is touching the kneecap. This ensures that both buttocks are placed firmly on the floor. ▶ Take the right elbow to the left side of the knee with the palm facing forward. Inhale and twist your spine, looking over your left shoulder. Keep your spine erect as you place your left hand to the floor for support. Exhale, breathe deeply and continue to stretch even further, holding for at least 10 seconds. Repeat to the other side. ▶ Sitting down on your heels, inhale and exhale slowly through the nose from the diaphragm for 10 seconds. Try to keep the breath rhythmic, deep, and even. ▶

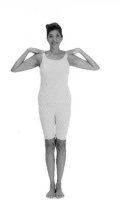
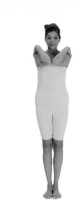

Day two
CIRCULATION

People who have good circulation feel robust, happy and healthy, while those with poor circulation may feel constantly depleted of energy and this affects their mental attitude. Fear of immobility and of growing old plagues even the happiest of people from time to time and so it is important to keep the body active and circulation flowing evenly. Poor circulation is a common complaint which can lead to various illnesses if not improved, so in this section I have designed a series of movements to boost your energy levels, raise your spirits and reoxygenate your entire system. You will notice that you are moving and twisting in every direction, which will stimulate all the internal organs and nerves, and combining this with deep breathing to release tension in the body.

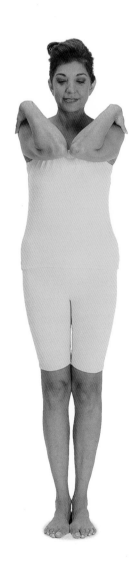

Stand with your feet together in perfect posture. Take your hands onto your shoulders, keeping the elbows up in a straight line to each other. ▸ Inhale and bring your elbows in towards each other. Exhale, and push the elbows back as far as possible to open the chest. ▸ Looking upwards, clasp your hands behind your head, lifting your elbows up as high as possible without lifting the shoulders. ▸ Inhale and bring your elbows towards each other, keeping your arms as close to the head as possible. ▸ Exhale and open your elbows wide, keeping your elbows in line and the shoulders down. ▸

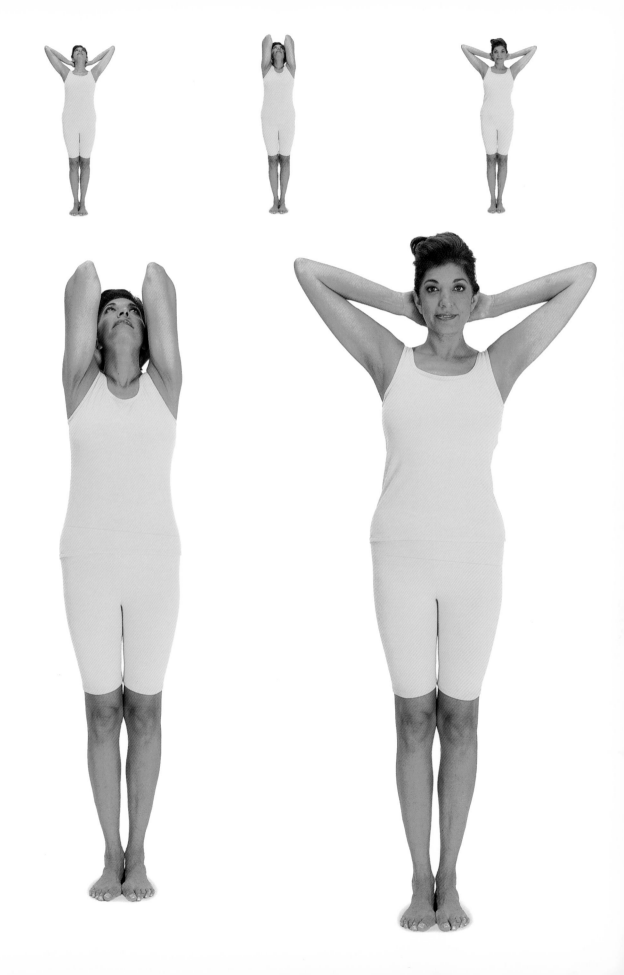

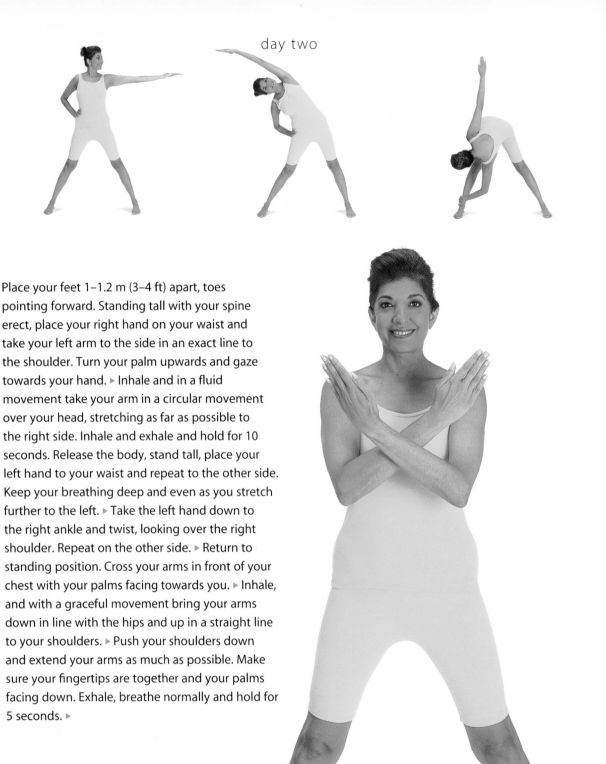

Place your feet 1–1.2 m (3–4 ft) apart, toes pointing forward. Standing tall with your spine erect, place your right hand on your waist and take your left arm to the side in an exact line to the shoulder. Turn your palm upwards and gaze towards your hand. ▸ Inhale and in a fluid movement take your arm in a circular movement over your head, stretching as far as possible to the right side. Inhale and exhale and hold for 10 seconds. Release the body, stand tall, place your left hand to your waist and repeat to the other side. Keep your breathing deep and even as you stretch further to the left. ▸ Take the left hand down to the right ankle and twist, looking over the right shoulder. Repeat on the other side. ▸ Return to standing position. Cross your arms in front of your chest with your palms facing towards you. ▸ Inhale, and with a graceful movement bring your arms down in line with the hips and up in a straight line to your shoulders. ▸ Push your shoulders down and extend your arms as much as possible. Make sure your fingertips are together and your palms facing down. Exhale, breathe normally and hold for 5 seconds. ▸

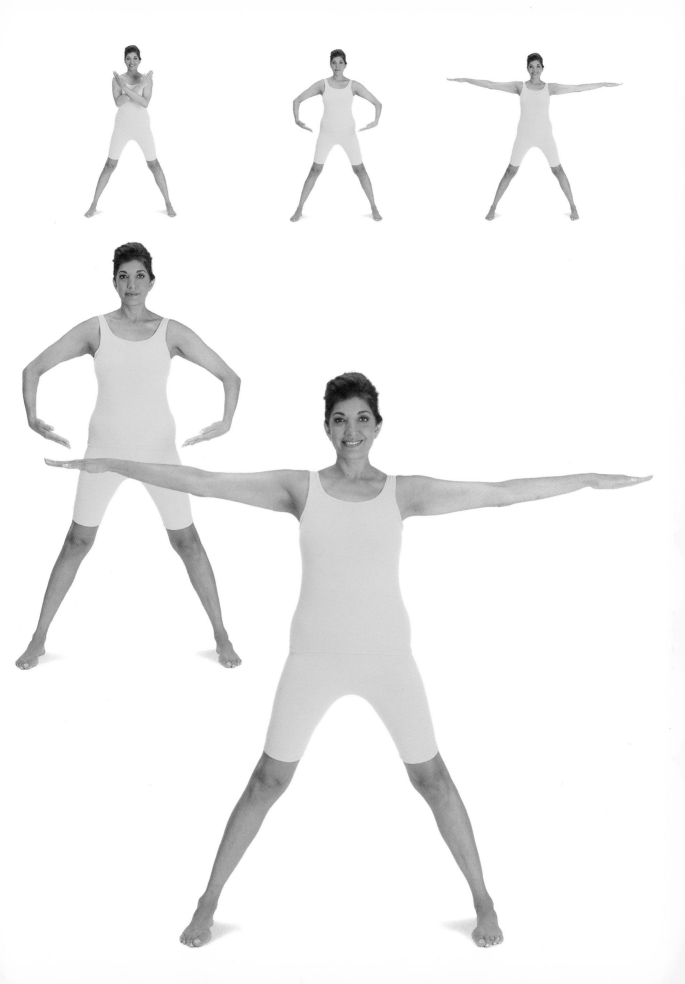

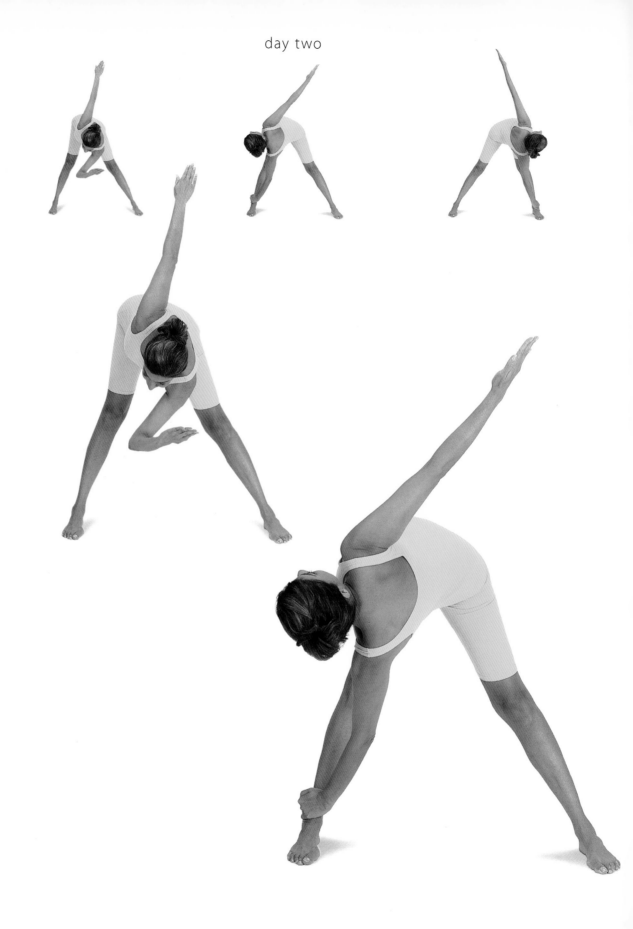

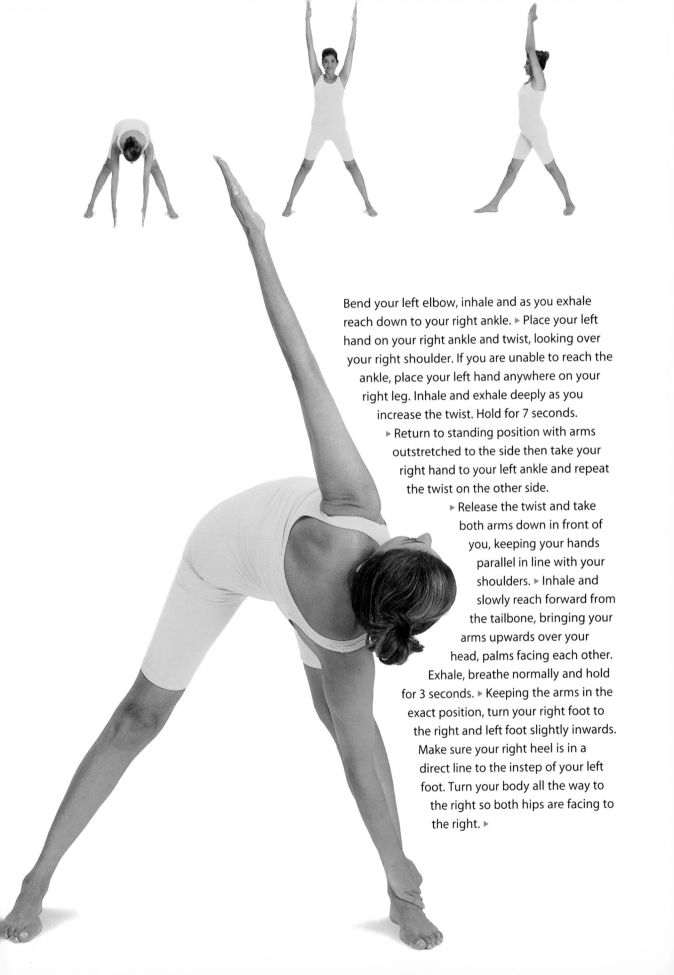

Bend your left elbow, inhale and as you exhale reach down to your right ankle. ▸ Place your left hand on your right ankle and twist, looking over your right shoulder. If you are unable to reach the ankle, place your left hand anywhere on your right leg. Inhale and exhale deeply as you increase the twist. Hold for 7 seconds.

▸ Return to standing position with arms outstretched to the side then take your right hand to your left ankle and repeat the twist on the other side.

▸ Release the twist and take both arms down in front of you, keeping your hands parallel in line with your shoulders. ▸ Inhale and slowly reach forward from the tailbone, bringing your arms upwards over your head, palms facing each other. Exhale, breathe normally and hold for 3 seconds. ▸ Keeping the arms in the exact position, turn your right foot to the right and left foot slightly inwards. Make sure your right heel is in a direct line to the instep of your left foot. Turn your body all the way to the right so both hips are facing to the right. ▸

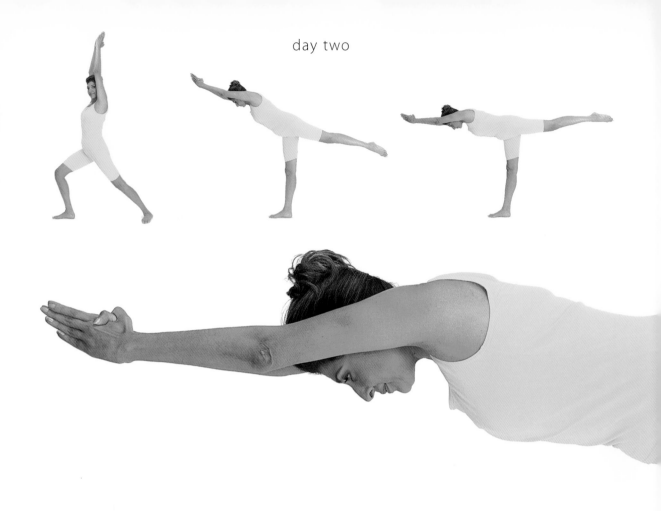

Bring your palms together in prayer position and cross your thumbs. Bend your right knee, making sure it does not overextend the right foot. ▸ Inhale, straighten your right leg and point your left foot as much as possible. This will help your left leg to remain straight. ▸ Exhale and lift your left leg up behind you, balancing on your right leg. Keep your arms in line to your head, close to your ears. Breathing deeply, continue to stretch in both directions so your spine is in a straight line to your arms and foot. Hold the position for 10 seconds and deepen the breath as the pose increases in intensity. ▸ To release, bend your right knee and take your left foot back to starting position. Straighten your right leg and place both hands

behind your lower back in prayer position, fingers pointing upwards. Inhale and take your head back, pushing your chest and hips forward. ▸ Exhale and, leading with the chin, stretch forward from the tailbone so your spine remains in a straight line. Breathe normally and hold for 5 seconds. ▸ Inhale, drop your head forward and stretch down towards your right knee. Exhale, breathe deeply and hold for 5 seconds. Inhale, release the spine and continue to stretch forward, keeping your spine straight. As you return to the starting position, push your hips forward and drop your head backwards. Exhale, breathe normally and straighten your spine. Repeat the entire exercise on the other side.

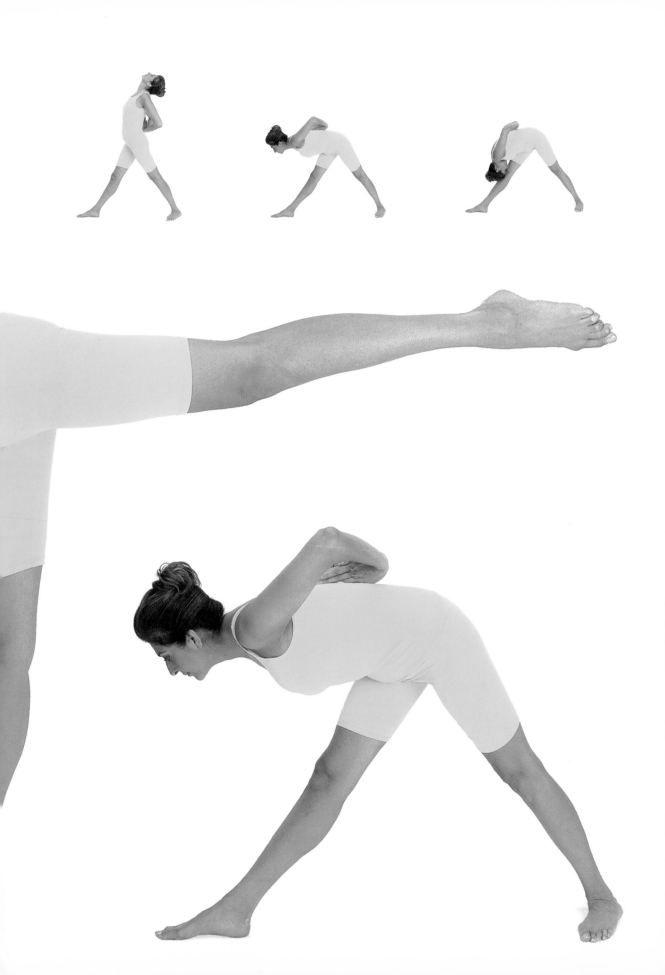

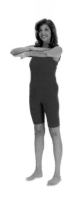
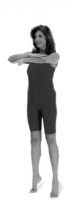

Day three
TONING

As we age our muscles begin to sag and it is vital to tone and strengthen them. Stretching is the best way to achieve top-to-toe fitness and yoga stretches the muscles lengthways, reducing the fat around each muscle and producing a long, lean, streamlined body. It also increases the flexibility and suppleness of the spine so that your movements are more fluid and graceful. A further benefit is that deep stretching stimulates lymphatic drainage which helps to eliminate cellulite, a common problem for women of all ages. The exercises in this section tone the areas of the body that show the signs of ageing first – legs, thighs, buttocks and tummies. The twisting movements help eliminate toxins from the system and the deep stretching movements increase circulation.

When toning the body it is very important to concentrate on the muscle groups you wish to firm. When you stand in perfect posture make sure every muscle in the body is working by lifting each muscle upwards, especially the muscle above the kneecap. Tighten your tummy muscles and tuck your tailbone under while you imagine a string pulling you upwards from the top of your head. Place your feet 30 cm (1 ft) apart, directly in line with your hips. Cross your arms in front of your chest, holding on to your elbows. ▶ Focus your attention on a spot in front of you. Rise up on your toes, lifting your heels up as high as possible.
▶ Now, keeping your spine in a straight line, bend your knees, lifting your heels up in a right angle to the floor. Hold the position, breathing deeply and evenly, for at least 10 seconds. You will find this position very challenging because you are combining balance with deep breathing. ▶ Now take the legs in a wide second position with your feet 1–1.2 m (3–4 ft) apart. Take your arms out to the side, in line with your shoulders. ▶ Turn your right foot to the right, making sure it is in an exact line to the instep of your left foot. Look over your right hand while keeping your spine upright. ▶

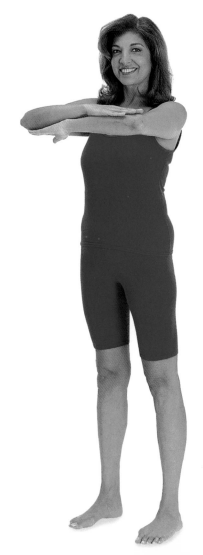

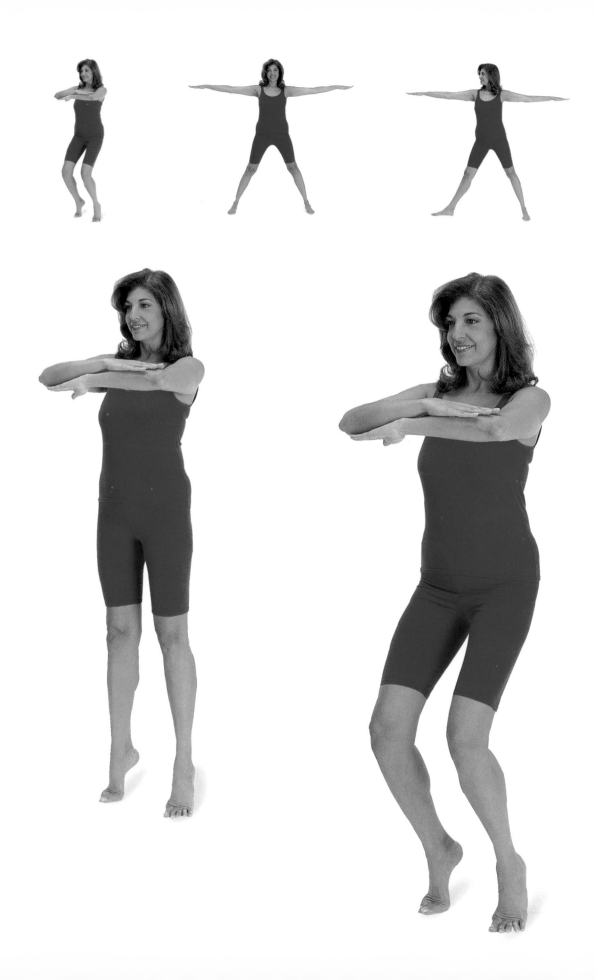

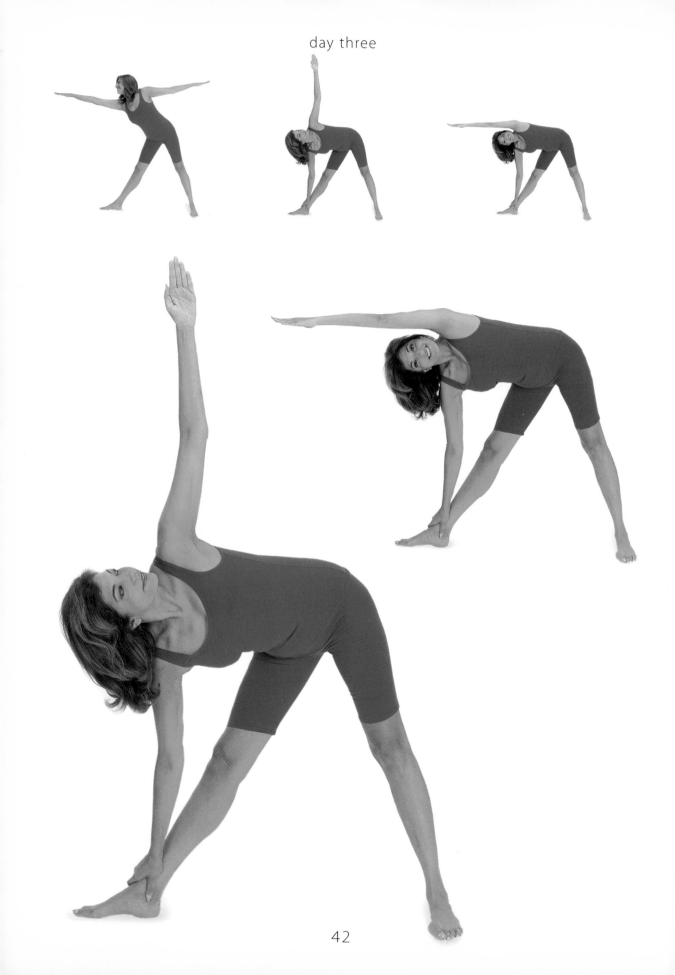

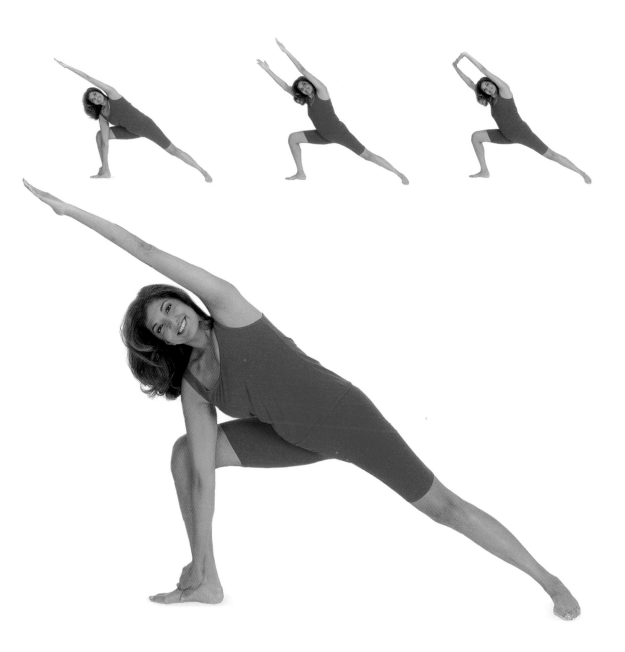

Leading from the tailbone, stretch out to the right as far as possible. ▸ Take your right hand down to your ankle and take your left arm upwards in a straight line. Make sure your fingertips are together and your palm is facing forward. Breathe deeply and normally as you hold for 7–10 seconds. ▸ Take your left arm over your head close to your ear in a straight line to the spine. Keep looking upwards as you inhale and exhale deeply for 10 seconds. ▸ Bend your right knee in an exact right angle so the back of the knee is in line to the right heel. Take your right palm to your instep and as you stretch diagonally take your left arm in an exact line to your left leg. Hold the pose for 10 seconds. ▸ Now take your right arm to join your left arm in a parallel line and hold the position while your breath deepens. Hold for 5 seconds. ▸ Clasp your hands together as you increase the stretch. Hold the position and breathe as deeply as possible for at least 10 seconds. ▸

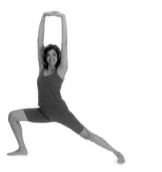
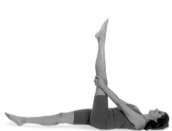
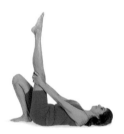

Lift your spine in a straight line as you clasp your hands over your head. Deepen the stretch as you lift your spine upwards to be as tall as possible. Inhale and straighten your knee and turn your body forward. Release your arms and take them to your sides. ▸ Lie back on the floor and relax your whole body, keeping your arms next to your body on either side. Inhale and lift your left leg upwards in an exact 90-degree angle to the floor. Clasp your hands together behind your knee and point your toes upwards. Hold for 5 seconds. ▸ Bend your right knee and bring your heel in as close to your right buttock as possible. ▸ Inhale and stretch your head to your left knee, keeping your leg in a straight line. Hold for 7 seconds, breathing deeply and evenly. Slowly lower your spine and then release your left leg down to the floor. Relax your right leg so both legs are down to the floor. Repeat the exercise on the other side. Inhale and exhale as you relax down. ▸ Bring both knees up, keeping your arms to your sides. ▸ Concentrate on your hips and tighten your buttock muscles as you lift your hips as high as possible. Breathing deeply, keep lifting the buttock muscles upwards. Hold your ankles if you are able to reach them – if not – hold anywhere along the leg that is comfortable. Draw your chin into your chest as you continue to lift your hips upwards. You are now in a perfect circular pose. To release, isolate the spine by pushing each vertebra down from the top of the spine so the tailbone is last to return to the floor. ▸

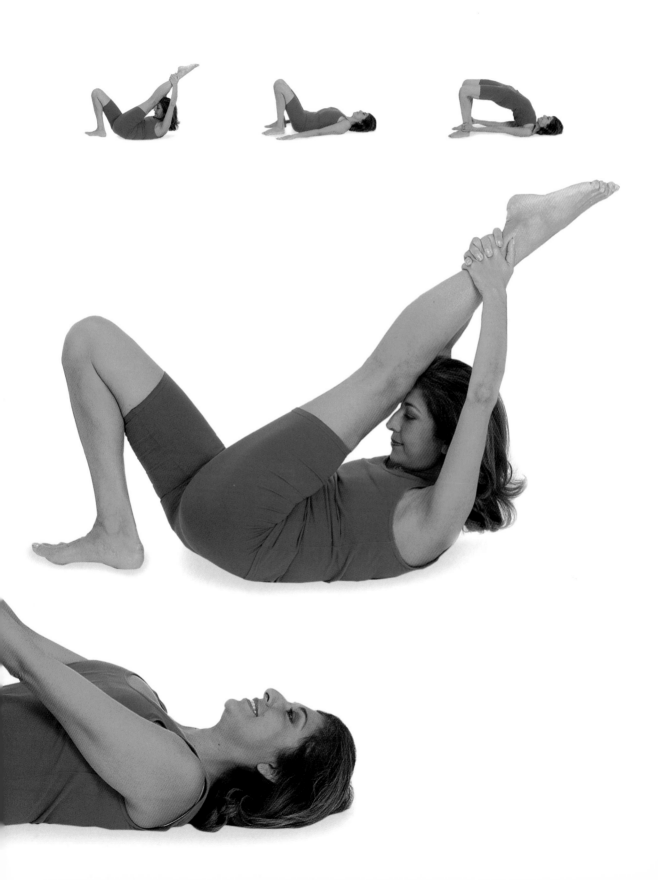

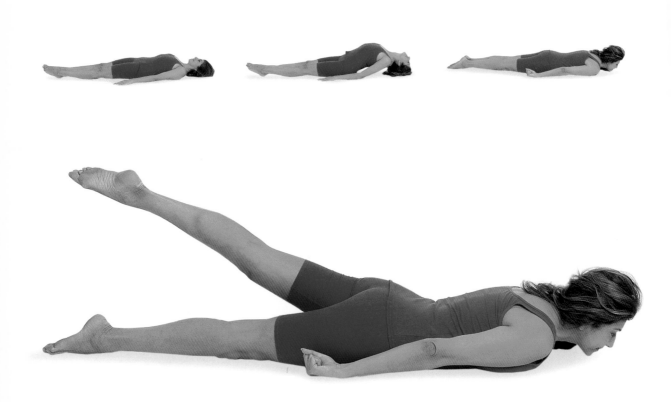

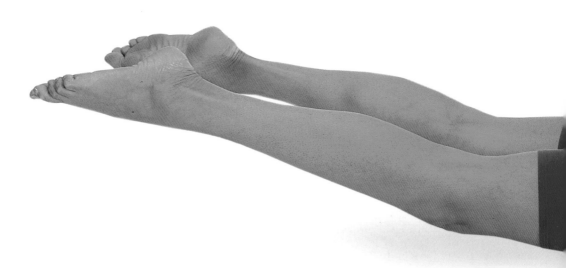

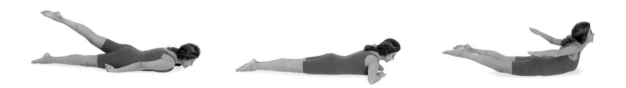

Release your hands from your ankles and relax your legs down to the floor. Inhale and exhale deeply for 5 seconds. ▸ Bring your legs together and point your toes down. Take your arms to your sides, palms on the floor. Inhale, push down on your elbows and raise your chest as high as possible so you are able to balance on the top of your head. Exhale, breathe normally and hold for 5–7 seconds. This is called the Fish pose and is an excellent stretch for the neck and chin. ▸ Turn over onto your stomach and place your chin on the floor. Place your hands in fists at your sides.

▸ Inhale, point your left foot to help straighten your knee and raise your left leg off the floor, keeping both hipbones down. Exhale, breathe normally and hold for 5–7 seconds. On an exhalation, slowly lower your leg. Repeat on the other side. ▸ Take your arms out to the side and rest on your elbows, fingers pointing inward. ▸ Inhale and simultaneously lift both legs and your chest off the floor, taking your arms behind you. Exhale, breathe deeply and hold for at least 10 seconds. This is an excellent exercise for toning and lifting the buttock muscles. Repeat and hold for 12–15 seconds.

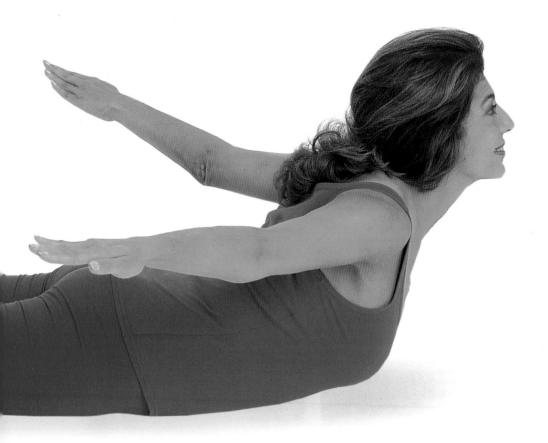

Day four
STRENGTHENING
THE BACK

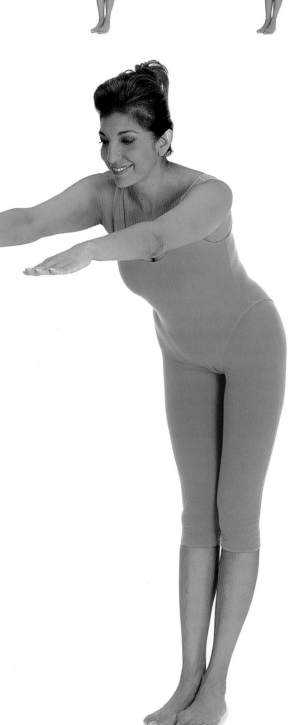

People who suffer from chronic back pain often believe that they should refrain from doing any exercise. In fact, it is vital to strengthen the muscles in the back to alleviate pain and prevent further back injuries. The exercises in this section are designed to eliminate the fear of moving the spine forwards and backwards. They will remove any muscular tension trapped in the back, relieve stiffness in the neck and shoulders and strengthen the muscles in the lower back to enable you to sit and stand in perfect posture. Pay special attention to all the muscles in the spine and perform slow, deliberate movements, taking deep and even breaths throughout. A dull pain in the spine merely indicates that your muscles are working, but if you feel any sharp pain stop the exercises immediately.

Stand with your feet together in perfect posture, arms to the side. Inhale and lift your arms up in front of you in line with your shoulders. Make sure your elbows are straight and your palms are facing down. Exhale, breathe normally and hold for 3 seconds. ▶ Concentrate on the area of the lower back and reach forward from the tailbone, keeping your spine straight and tightening your tummy muscles as you stretch down. ▶ Using the natural body weight combined with deep inhalations and exhalations to loosen the spine, stretch right down so your hands reach the floor. Do not force or jerk your body down. You will be surprised how supple

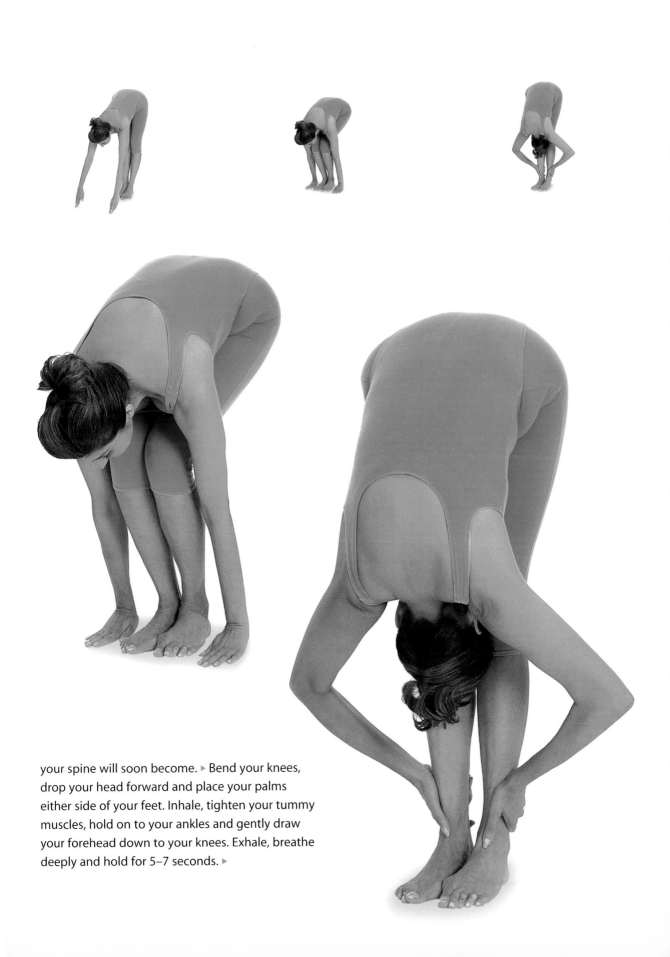

your spine will soon become. ▸ Bend your knees, drop your head forward and place your palms either side of your feet. Inhale, tighten your tummy muscles, hold on to your ankles and gently draw your forehead down to your knees. Exhale, breathe deeply and hold for 5–7 seconds. ▸

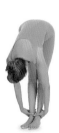 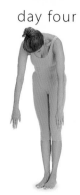 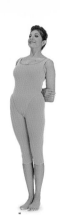

Release your hands and begin to uncurl your spine slowly, keeping your knees straight. ▸ Pull your tummy muscles up, tighten your buttock muscles, drop your shoulders and lift your head up. ▸ When you are standing tall, take both arms behind your lower back, holding firmly on to your elbows. ▸ Inhale and push your hips forward as much as possible. Keep your knees straight, open your chest and drop your head back. Exhale, breathe normally and relax your neck and jaw. Hold for 5–7 seconds. Slowly release by returning to standing position and relax forward to counteract the back bend. ▸ Relax down to the floor with your legs outstretched in front and arms to the side. Inhale, point your toes and bring your knees into your chest. Stretch your arms out in line with your shoulders. ▸ Exhale and take both knees to the right as you twist your spine to the left side and look over your left shoulder. ▸

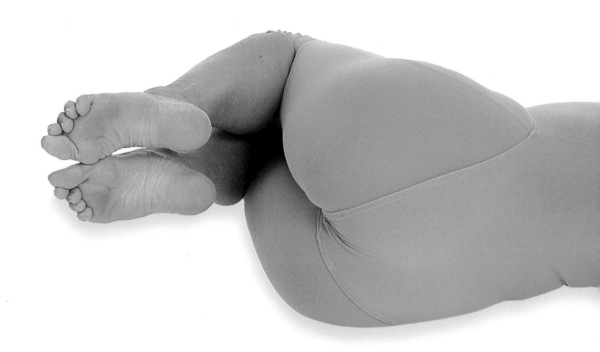

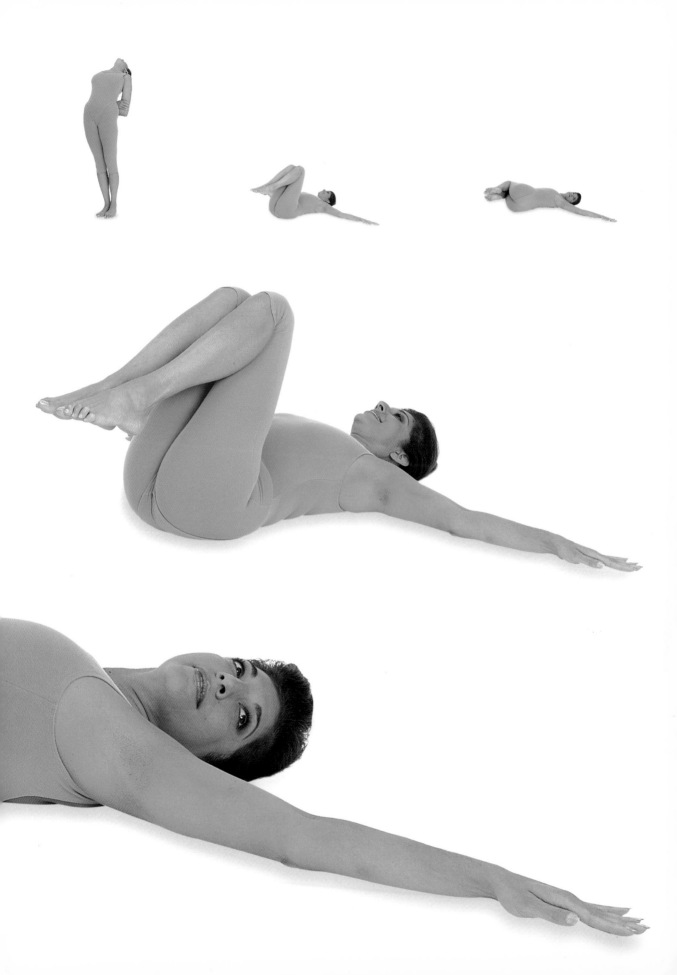

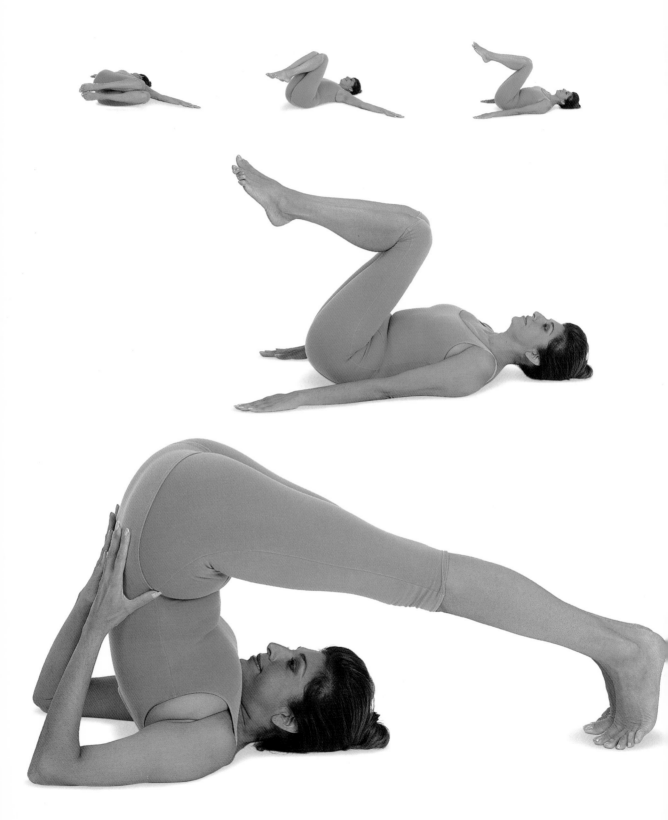

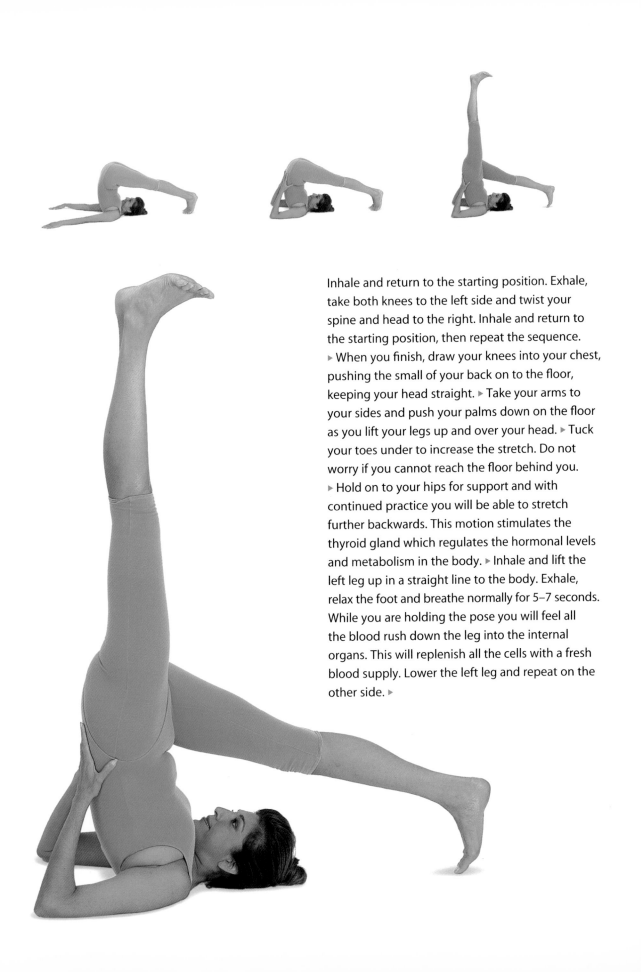

Inhale and return to the starting position. Exhale, take both knees to the left side and twist your spine and head to the right. Inhale and return to the starting position, then repeat the sequence. ▸ When you finish, draw your knees into your chest, pushing the small of your back on to the floor, keeping your head straight. ▸ Take your arms to your sides and push your palms down on the floor as you lift your legs up and over your head. ▸ Tuck your toes under to increase the stretch. Do not worry if you cannot reach the floor behind you. ▸ Hold on to your hips for support and with continued practice you will be able to stretch further backwards. This motion stimulates the thyroid gland which regulates the hormonal levels and metabolism in the body. ▸ Inhale and lift the left leg up in a straight line to the body. Exhale, relax the foot and breathe normally for 5–7 seconds. While you are holding the pose you will feel all the blood rush down the leg into the internal organs. This will replenish all the cells with a fresh blood supply. Lower the left leg and repeat on the other side. ▸

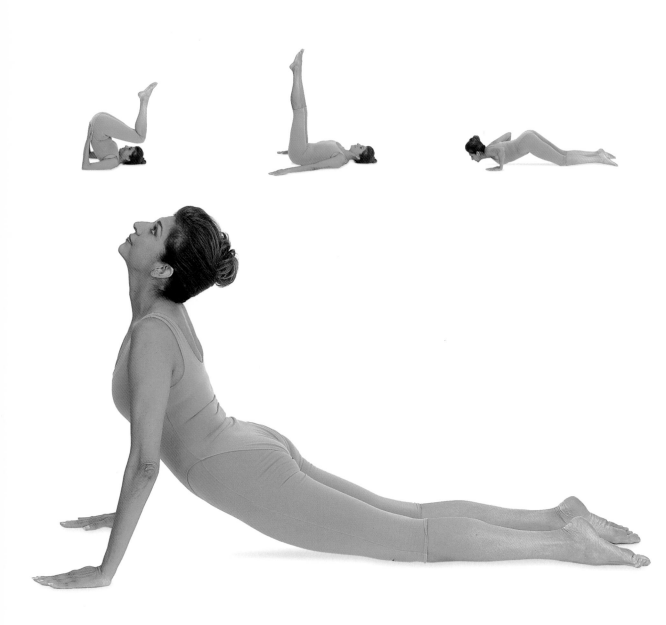

Slowly bend both legs and lower your knees to your forehead. ▸ When you reach a 90-degree angle to the floor, straighten your legs and hold the position, breathing deeply and evenly, for 10 seconds. Using the tummy muscles, slowly lower your legs to the floor. Relax. ▸ Turn over, place your hands directly under your shoulders and push your hips back so you are sitting on your heels. Stretch your arms out in front. Inhale and dive forward with your chest so your hips are up and your chest is in line with your head. ▸ In a circular motion, lift your spine and look upwards as you balance on your hands. ▸ Relax down to the floor. Bend both knees and take hold of your ankles. Place your chin on the floor. ▸ Inhale, lift your legs and head and balance on your hipbones. Exhale, then breathe deeply and evenly as you continue to stretch upwards. Hold for 5 seconds then release slowly.

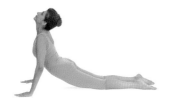
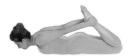

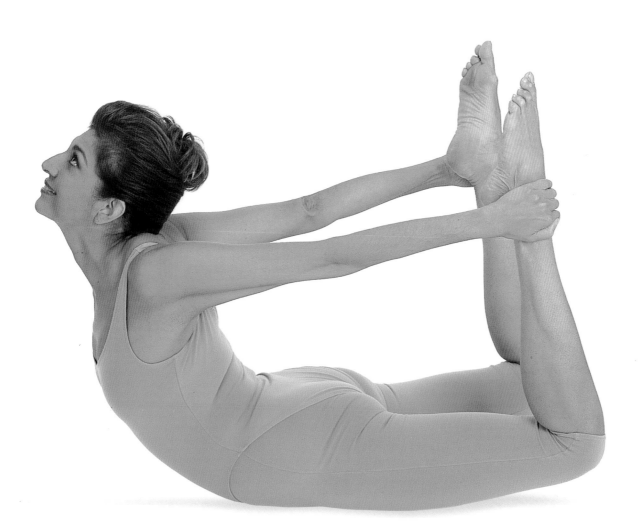

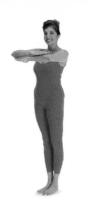
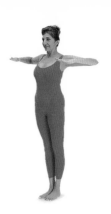

Day five
OPENING THE
CHEST

In yoga there are considered to be seven energy centres, or chakras, which relate to different parts of the body. These spinning wheels of energy must be flowing smoothly and evenly before a person can be truly balanced and centered, and this can only occur when the mind, body and soul are in total harmony and balance. The fifth chakra is related to the heart, which controls loving emotions. People who have suffered bad experiences will tend to close their heart to protect themselves from further pain. Opening the chest will help you to gain a more positive outlook on life in general; you will feel empowered and have the confidence to face the world with a brave heart.

Stand tall with your feet together. Take your arms up in front of your chest and bend your elbows, placing the right forearm over the left. Keep your arms level with your shoulders. ▸ Inhale, take your elbows back and open your chest. You will feel your shoulderblades moving towards each other. Exhale and return to the starting position. Repeat the exercise. ▸ Release your elbows and take your forearms in front of you in a parallel line with the palms facing towards each other. ▸ Inhale and take your elbows back as far as possible, palms facing forward. Exhale and return to the starting position. Repeat. ▸ Stand in perfect posture. Lift your chest upwards while keeping your shoulders down. Inhale and lift your left knee up. Exhale, clasp both hands around your knee and draw your leg closer to your body. Breathing deeply, hold for 5 seconds. If you are unable to balance, lean your back against a wall or use a chair for assistance. ▸

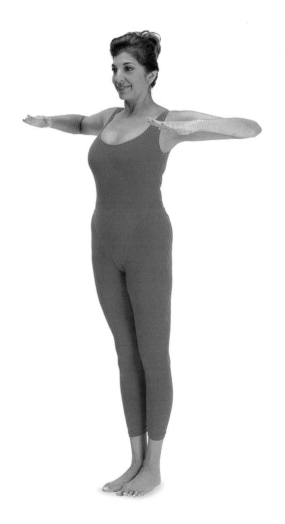

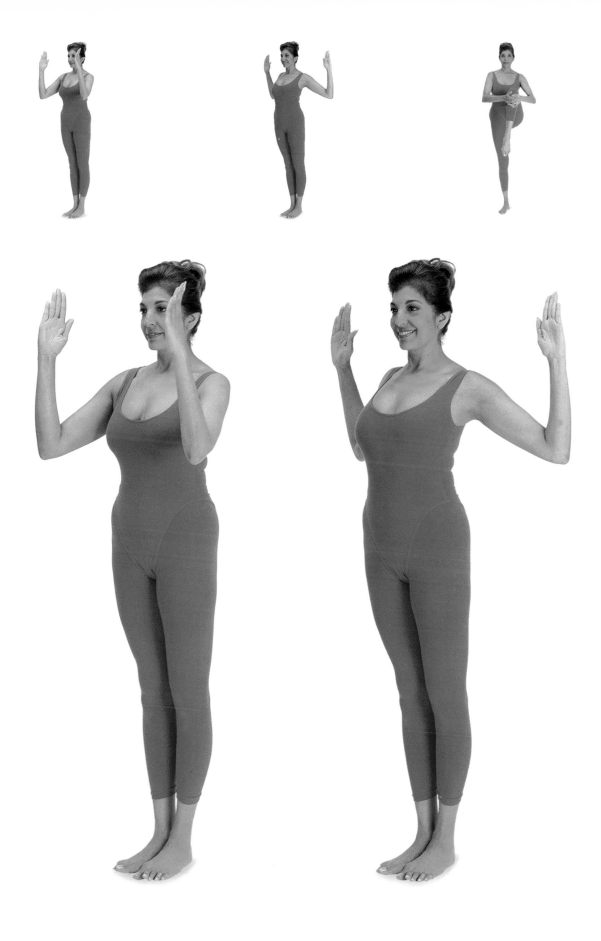

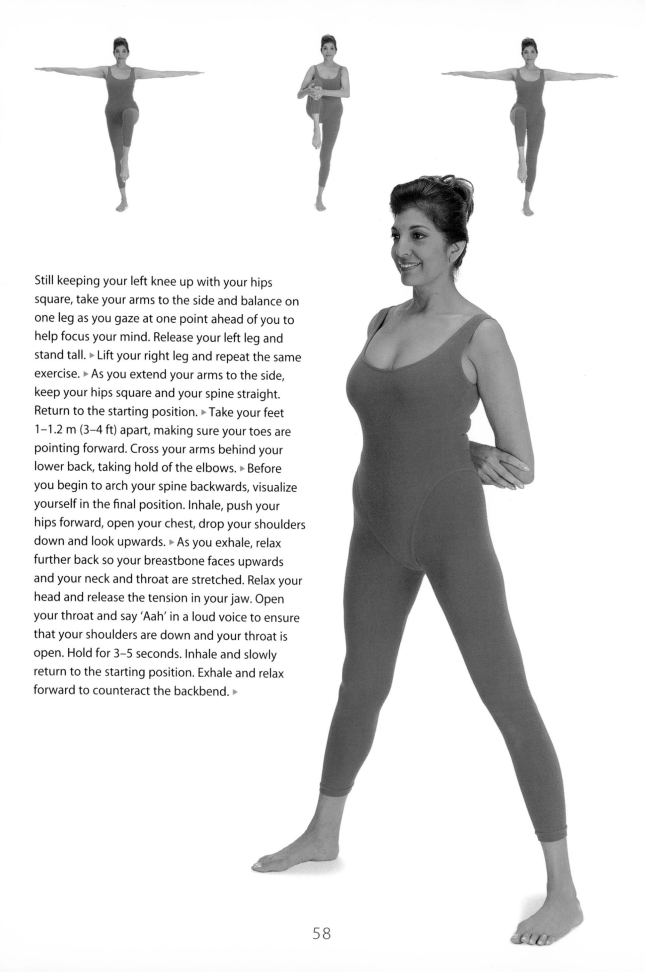

Still keeping your left knee up with your hips square, take your arms to the side and balance on one leg as you gaze at one point ahead of you to help focus your mind. Release your left leg and stand tall. ▸ Lift your right leg and repeat the same exercise. ▸ As you extend your arms to the side, keep your hips square and your spine straight. Return to the starting position. ▸ Take your feet 1–1.2 m (3–4 ft) apart, making sure your toes are pointing forward. Cross your arms behind your lower back, taking hold of the elbows. ▸ Before you begin to arch your spine backwards, visualize yourself in the final position. Inhale, push your hips forward, open your chest, drop your shoulders down and look upwards. ▸ As you exhale, relax further back so your breastbone faces upwards and your neck and throat are stretched. Relax your head and release the tension in your jaw. Open your throat and say 'Aah' in a loud voice to ensure that your shoulders are down and your throat is open. Hold for 3–5 seconds. Inhale and slowly return to the starting position. Exhale and relax forward to counteract the backbend. ▸

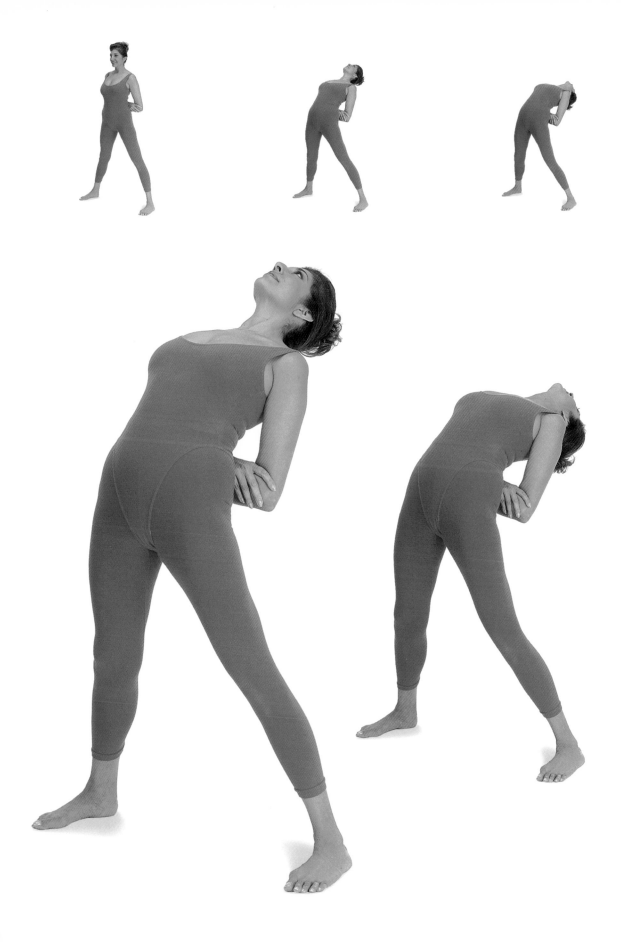

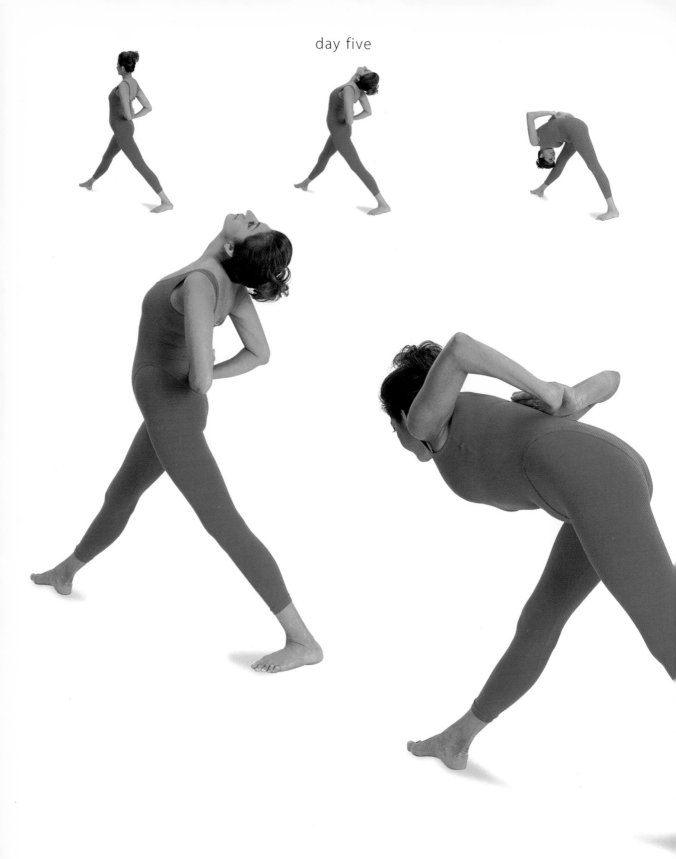

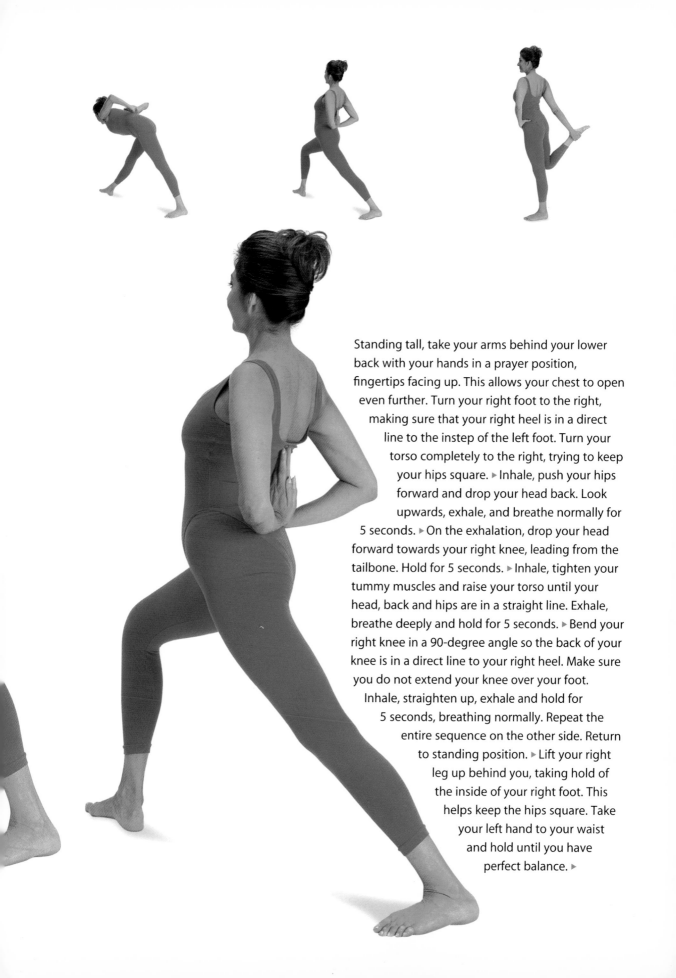

Standing tall, take your arms behind your lower back with your hands in a prayer position, fingertips facing up. This allows your chest to open even further. Turn your right foot to the right, making sure that your right heel is in a direct line to the instep of the left foot. Turn your torso completely to the right, trying to keep your hips square. ▸ Inhale, push your hips forward and drop your head back. Look upwards, exhale, and breathe normally for 5 seconds. ▸ On the exhalation, drop your head forward towards your right knee, leading from the tailbone. Hold for 5 seconds. ▸ Inhale, tighten your tummy muscles and raise your torso until your head, back and hips are in a straight line. Exhale, breathe deeply and hold for 5 seconds. ▸ Bend your right knee in a 90-degree angle so the back of your knee is in a direct line to your right heel. Make sure you do not extend your knee over your foot. Inhale, straighten up, exhale and hold for 5 seconds, breathing normally. Repeat the entire sequence on the other side. Return to standing position. ▸ Lift your right leg up behind you, taking hold of the inside of your right foot. This helps keep the hips square. Take your left hand to your waist and hold until you have perfect balance. ▸

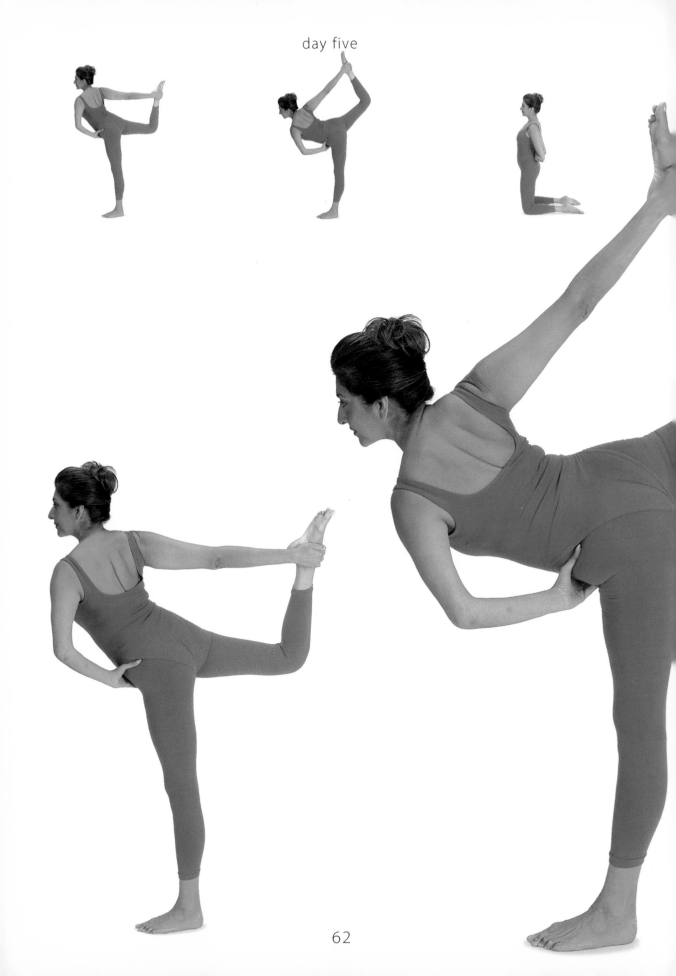

62

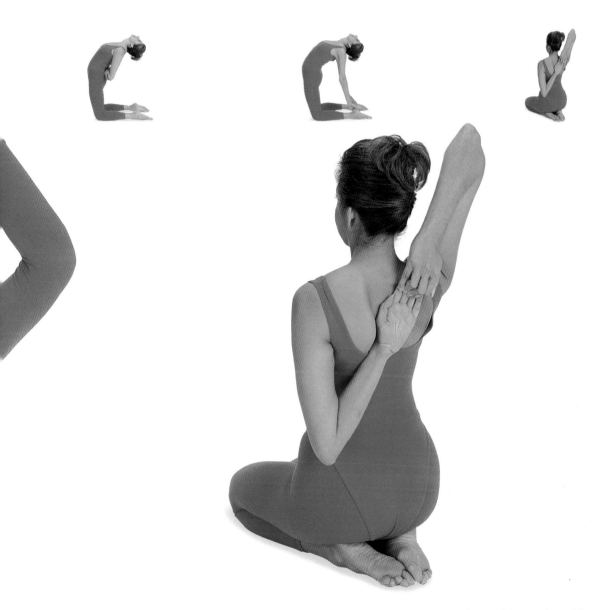

Focus your attention on a spot in front of you and begin to raise your right leg. ▶ Maintaining your balance, stretch even further, pointing your toe. Breathing deeply, hold for as long as possible, stretching in both directions. Repeat on the other side. ▶ Kneel on the floor, your knees in a direct line to your hips and arms behind your lower back. ▶ Pushing from your hips, arch backwards. ▶ If you can, place your hands on your heels to increase the stretch. Continue to push your hips up, breathing deeply, and hold for 5–7 seconds. ▶ Sit on your heels and drop your head forward to counteract the pose. Lift your head and take your right arm over your right shoulder so your palm is facing your right shoulderblade. Take your left arm behind your back, palm facing outward. Inhale and try to clasp the palms together. Exhale, breathe normally and hold for 6 seconds. Repeat on the other side.

Day six
OPENING THE HIPS

In yoga the weight of the body is used to release and open tight areas. Never force your body – use deep breathing instead. Opening the hips and allowing the thighs to rotate outwards has enormous benefits for the whole body: posture is improved, ligaments are loosened and a more balanced spine is achieved. Also, opening the groin will allow the blood to move more freely through the body, increasing the supply to the heart. Only when the hip area is totally opened will you be able to sit comfortably in the full lotus position. Yogis always meditate in a lotus position because their tailbone is able to touch the floor, connecting the chakras to the ground. As you inhale, the breath enters the lower abdomen which connects with the tailbone or first chakra and moves up through the spine to the seventh or crown chakra. This continuous flow of energy raises the level of consciousness.

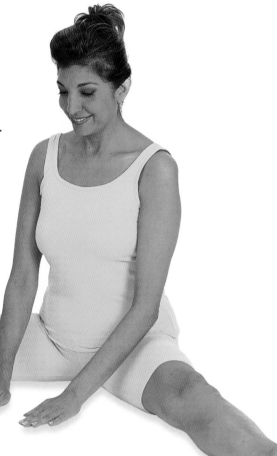

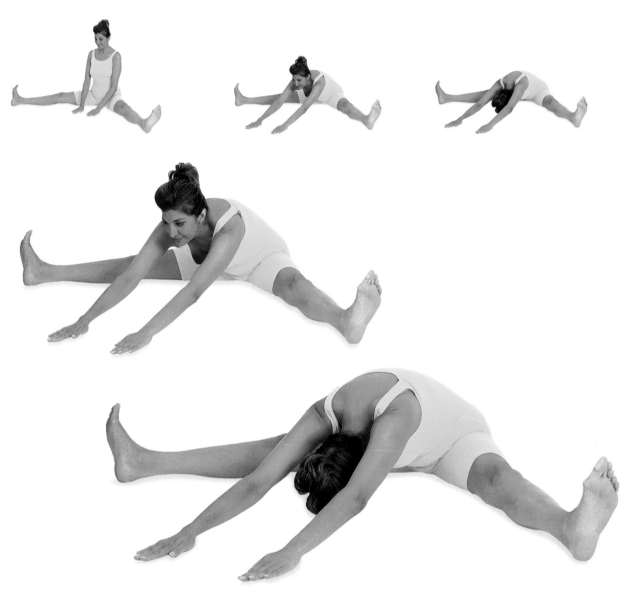

Sit up tall with your legs outstretched in front of you. Bend your knees and bring the soles of your feet together. Lean forward, hold on to your ankles and draw your heels in towards your pubic bone as close as possible. You will find that both knees are off the floor; do not try to bounce them down to the floor as this jars the hip joints and actually causes extra stiffness to the hips. ▸ In order to open the hips, breathe deeply and evenly while you relax your head over your feet. Hold for at least 10–15 seconds. ▸ Slowly uncurl your spine and sit in perfect posture. Take your legs wide apart. Rotate your knees outward, flex your toes so the backs of your knees reach the floor and place your palms on the floor. ▸ Inhale and stretch your arms forward as much as possible. ▸ Exhale and drop your head forward. Breathe deeply and evenly as you relax down further. Hold for 10–15 seconds. ▸

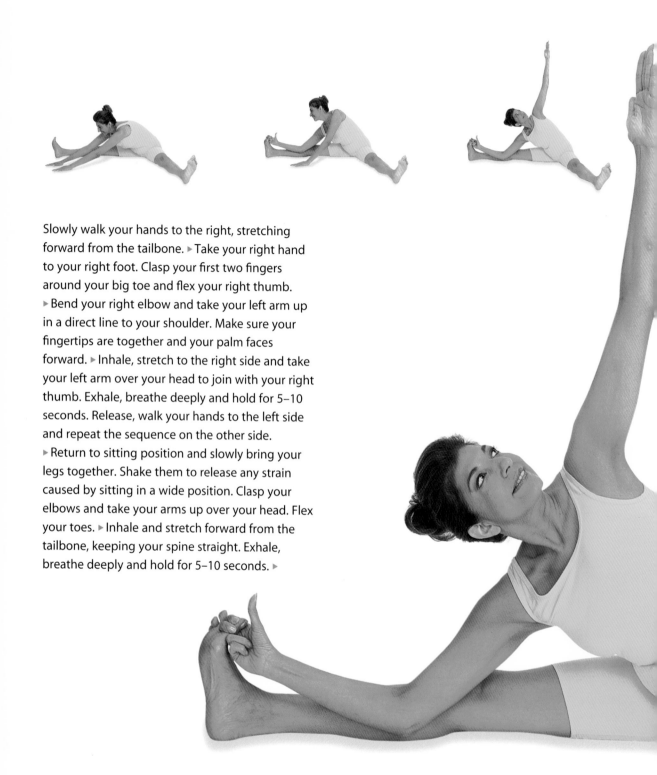

Slowly walk your hands to the right, stretching forward from the tailbone. ▸ Take your right hand to your right foot. Clasp your first two fingers around your big toe and flex your right thumb. ▸ Bend your right elbow and take your left arm up in a direct line to your shoulder. Make sure your fingertips are together and your palm faces forward. ▸ Inhale, stretch to the right side and take your left arm over your head to join with your right thumb. Exhale, breathe deeply and hold for 5–10 seconds. Release, walk your hands to the left side and repeat the sequence on the other side. ▸ Return to sitting position and slowly bring your legs together. Shake them to release any strain caused by sitting in a wide position. Clasp your elbows and take your arms up over your head. Flex your toes. ▸ Inhale and stretch forward from the tailbone, keeping your spine straight. Exhale, breathe deeply and hold for 5–10 seconds. ▸

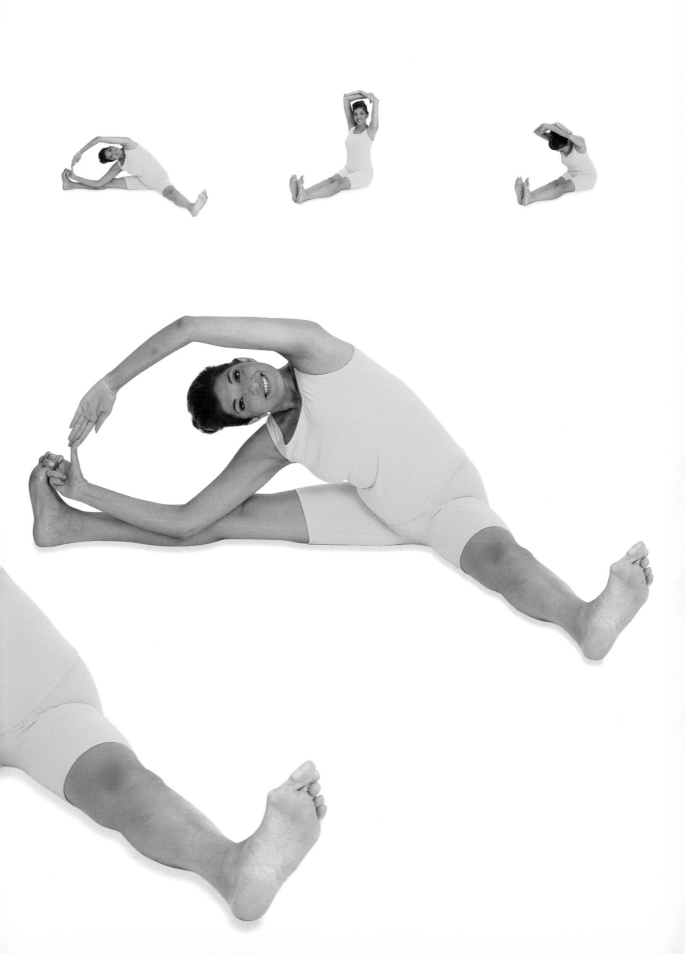

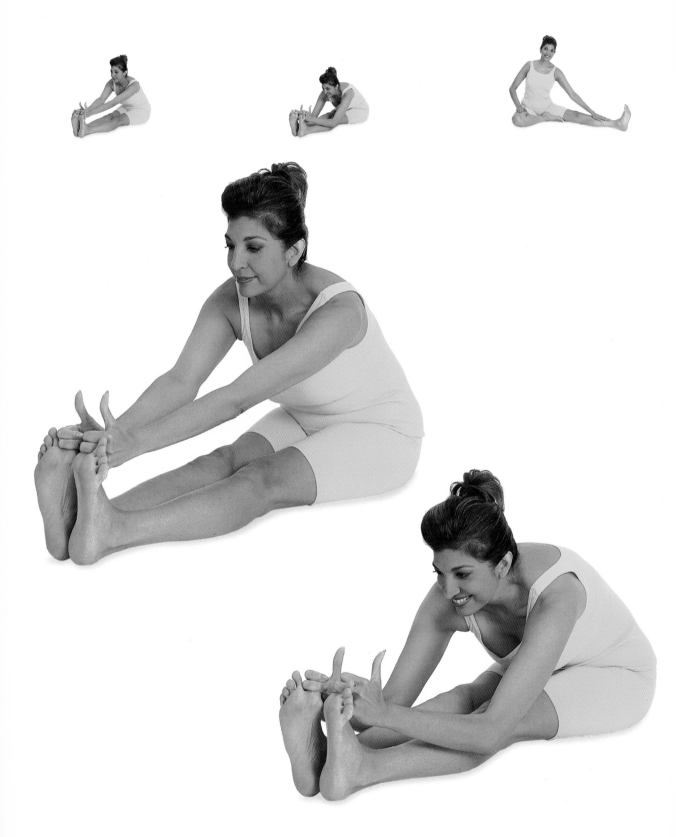

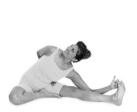 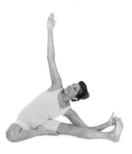 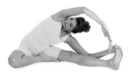

Reaching forward from the tailbone, clasp the two first fingers around your big toes and flex your thumbs back. ▸ Inhale, tighten the tummy and stretch forward, drawing the elbows to the floor. Exhale. Breathing deeply and evenly, hold for 10 seconds. ▸ Inhale, slowly uncurl your spine and sit up tall. Exhale. Bring your right leg up to the inner thigh. Try to place your right knee on the floor. Place your left hand on your calf and your right hand on your thigh close to the knee. ▸ Take your right arm behind your back and twist, looking over your right shoulder as you drop your left elbow to the floor. Clasp your first two fingers around your big toe and flex your thumb. Breathing deeply and evenly, hold for 7–10 seconds. ▸ Release your right arm and bring it up in line with your shoulder, fingers together, palm forward. ▸ Inhale, stretch to the left and touch the fingertips and thumb together. Repeat on the other side. ▸

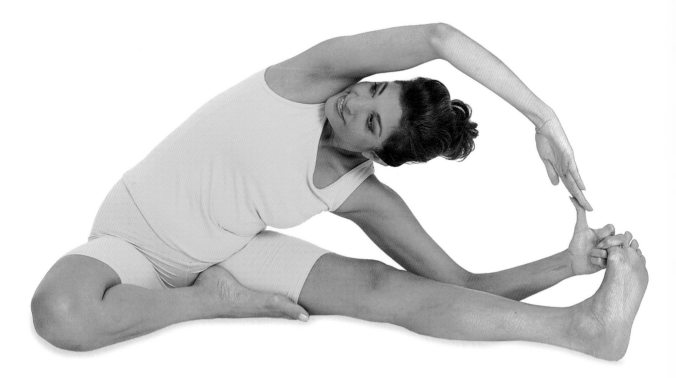

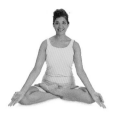 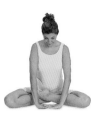 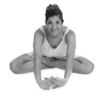

Sit up tall in a comfortable cross-legged position. Open your hands, place the first finger and thumb together and extend the remaining fingertips down towards the floor. Concentrating on the diaphragm, inhale and exhale deeply for 10 seconds, remembering that as you inhale the tummy is extended outwards and as you exhale the tummy comes in. ▶ Place your palms on the floor, interlace your fingers and gaze down at your hands. ▶ Inhale and stretch forward from the tailbone, reaching your arms out as far as possible in front of you. ▶ Exhale and take your arms in a circular motion over your head. Sit up tall, drop your head back and look up at your hands. Breathing normally, hold for 5–7 seconds. ▶ Lift your head, keeping your arms close to your ears. Turn your body towards your left knee. ▶ Inhale, and as you exhale stretch your arms down to the floor as you drop your head to your knee. Breathe deeply and evenly and hold for 7–10 seconds. Inhale, sit up tall and exhale. Repeat on the other side.

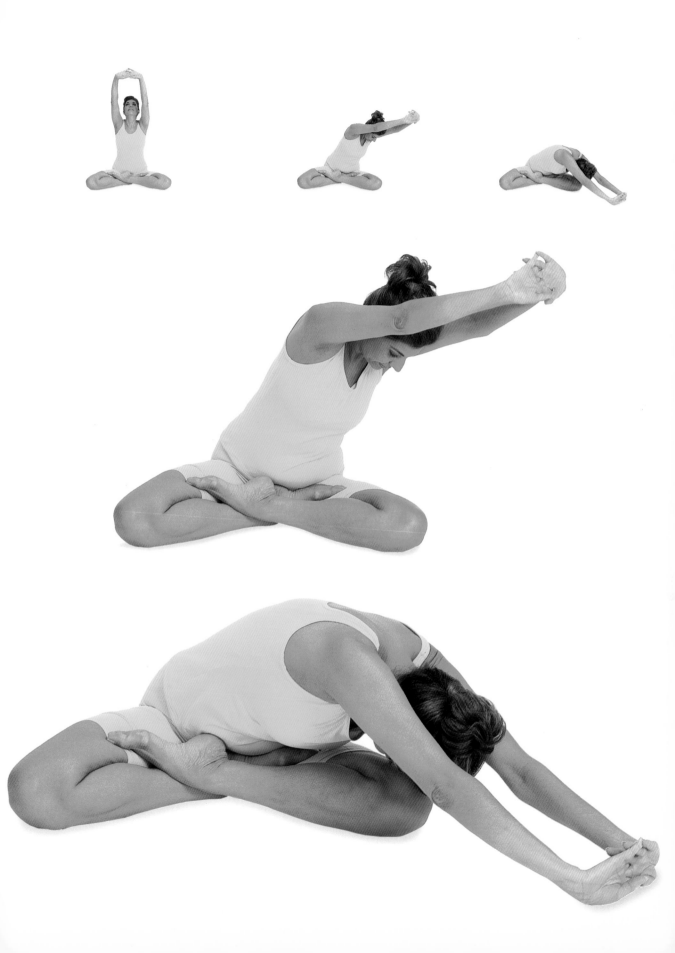

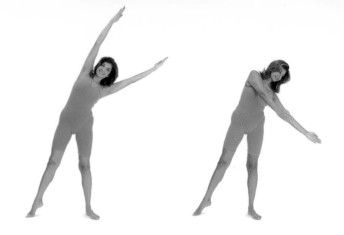

Day seven
ENERGIZING

Yoga is a form of exercise which constantly builds energy levels rather than depleting them. With advancing age there comes a drop in energy and some people believe that they should not do any form of exercise. Harsh and strenuous movements are harmful at any age but because yoga is very gentle on the joints even the very elderly can benefit. Try to keep the movements fluid and allow your whole body to move gracefully like a dancer. If you become short of breath during the series take deeper breaths from the diaphragm to increase your energy flow. Repeat the section at least twice to feel the benefit and, at the end, bring your fingertips together to feel an exchange of energy from your right hand to your left.

This series of movements will energize your entire system, especially if you are feeling tired and lack energy to enjoy the pastimes you enjoy most. As you age it is more important to feel enthusiastic and full of vitality. Stand tall with your feet 1–1.2 m (3–4 ft) apart. Shift your weight to the left foot, lift the right heel off the floor and point the right foot and take both arms to the left. Extend your arms, palms facing each other, and stretch your body up, lifting your chest. ▶ Inhale and begin to swing your arms to the left in a wide circle. ▶ Bend your knees to increase the movement and take your arms down in front of you in a parallel line. ▶ Continue to swing your arms to the right and shift your weight to the right foot. ▶ As you bring your arms over to the left, exhale, and swing your body simultaneously to the left, completing the full circle. To increase the stretch take the left arm out to the side. ▶

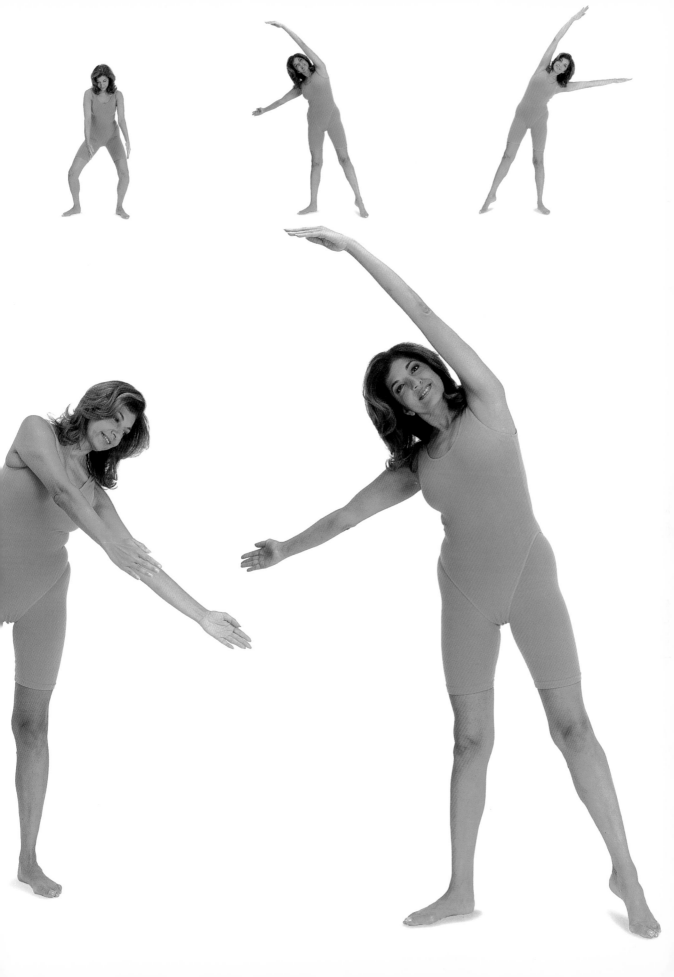

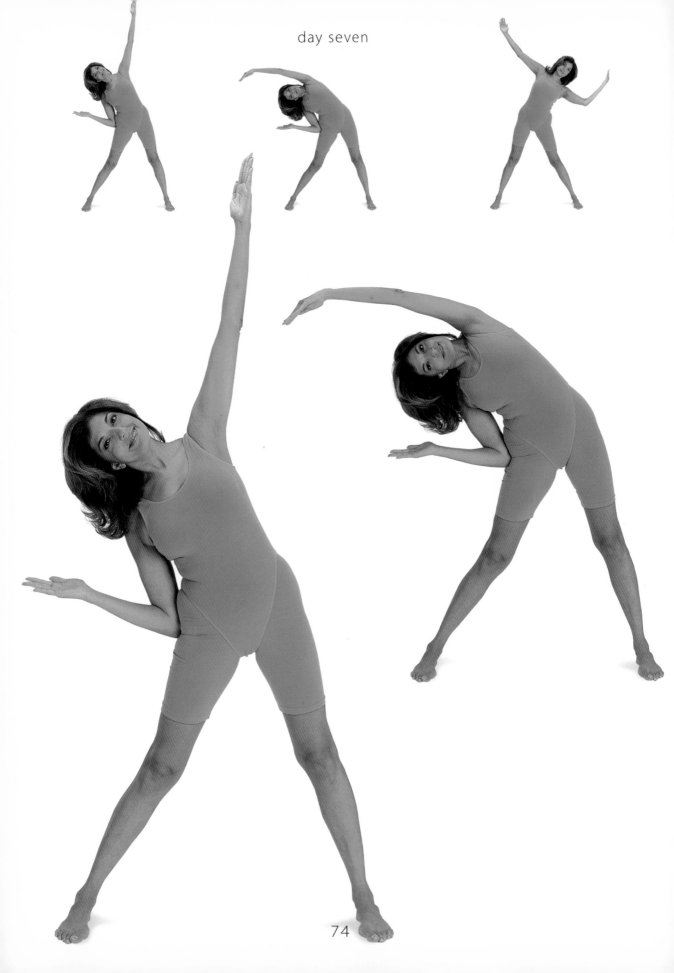

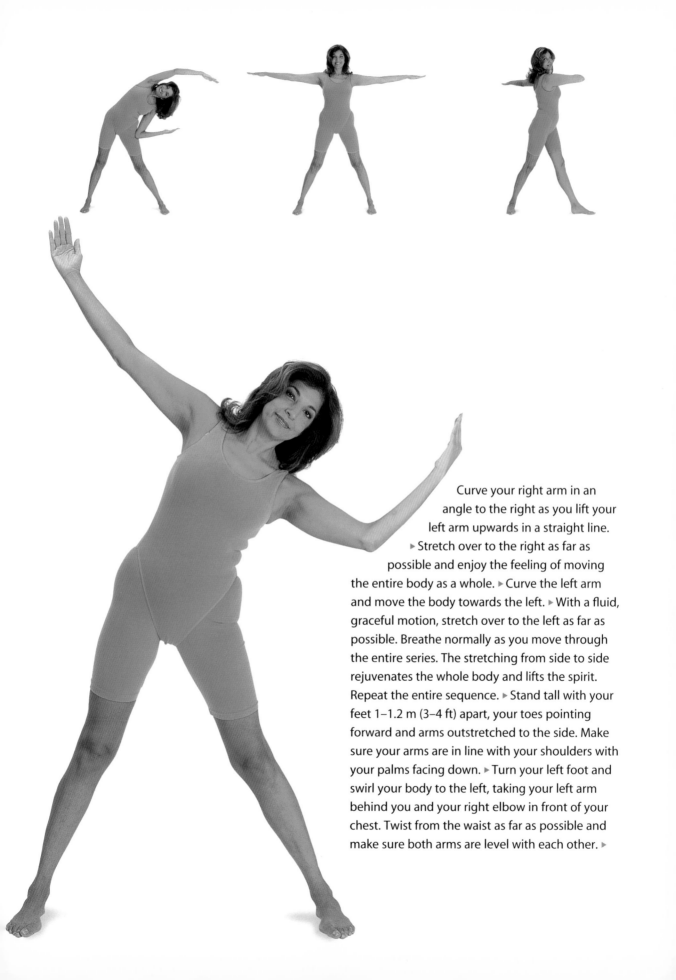

Curve your right arm in an angle to the right as you lift your left arm upwards in a straight line. ▸ Stretch over to the right as far as possible and enjoy the feeling of moving the entire body as a whole. ▸ Curve the left arm and move the body towards the left. ▸ With a fluid, graceful motion, stretch over to the left as far as possible. Breathe normally as you move through the entire series. The stretching from side to side rejuvenates the whole body and lifts the spirit. Repeat the entire sequence. ▸ Stand tall with your feet 1–1.2 m (3–4 ft) apart, your toes pointing forward and arms outstretched to the side. Make sure your arms are in line with your shoulders with your palms facing down. ▸ Turn your left foot and swirl your body to the left, taking your left arm behind you and your right elbow in front of your chest. Twist from the waist as far as possible and make sure both arms are level with each other. ▸

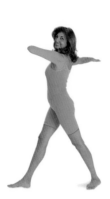

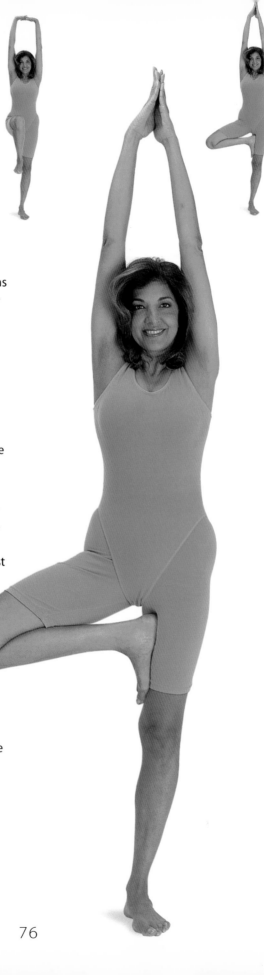

Turn your right foot and swing your body and arms to the right. Return to standing position with your feet together. ▸ Keeping both hips square, raise your right knee and balance on your left foot. When you have perfect balance raise both arms over your head. Clasp your hands together and hold the position for 5 seconds. ▸ Breathing normally, take your right leg up and place your right foot on the inside of your left thigh. Make sure the standing leg is straight and lift the muscle above the kneecap to help you balance. Stretch your arms over your head, keeping your elbows straight. Cross your thumbs and place your palms together. Hold for 5 seconds. ▸ Release your arms, place your left hand on your waist and take your right hand down to your right foot. Clasp your first and second fingers around your big toe and flex your thumb. As you grab hold of your foot lean towards the right, keeping your spine erect. ▸ Inhale and stretch your leg out to the side as far as possible. Exhale, breathe normally and hold for 5 seconds. If you cannot extend the right leg fully, do not worry – it is more important to keep the hips square and the standing leg straight. ▸ Release your leg and place your feet 1–1.2 m (3–4 ft) apart. Turn your right foot to the right and bend your right knee. Place your hand on top of your knee with your fingers facing the inner thigh. ▸

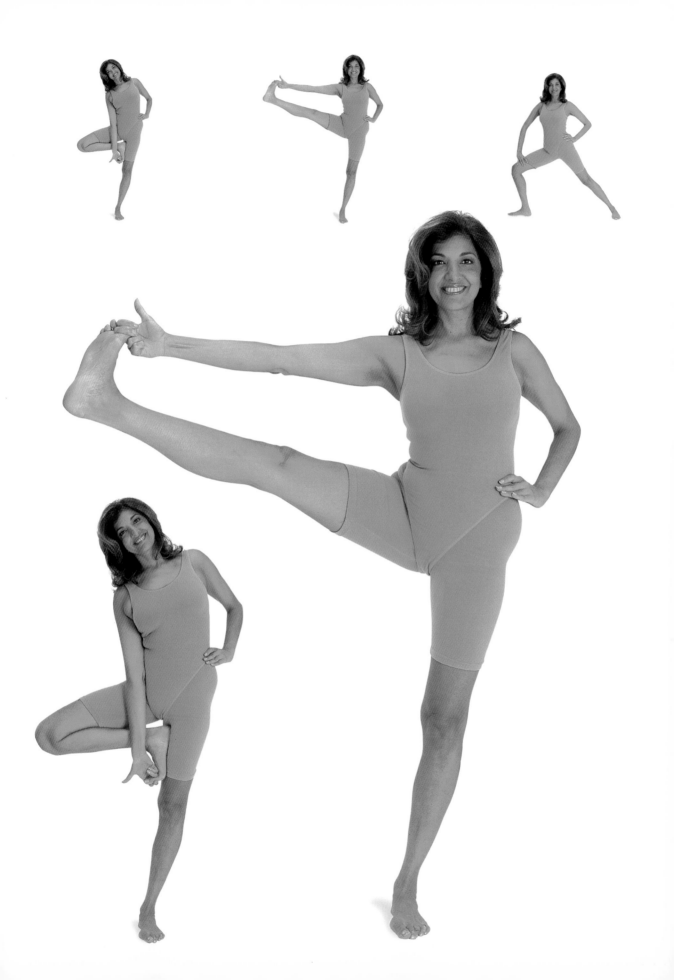

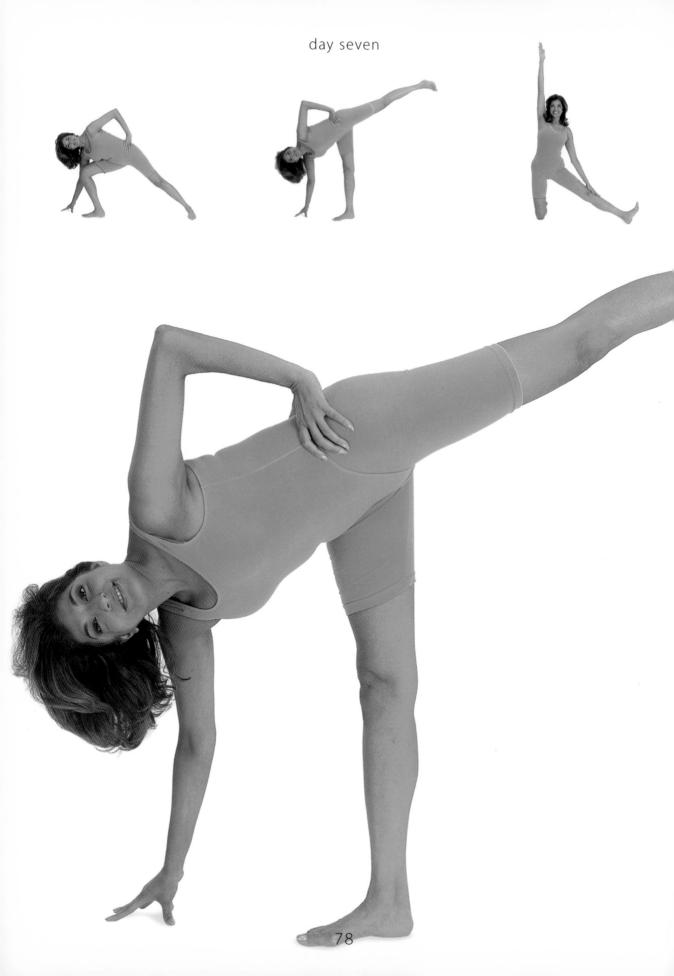

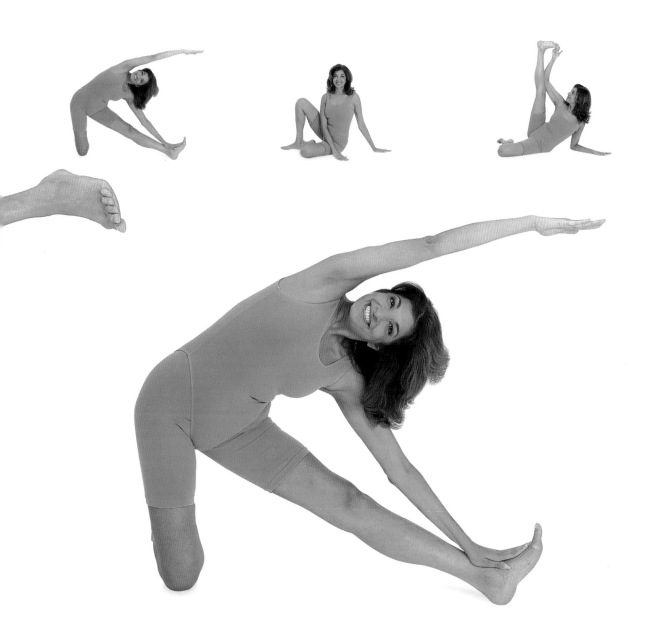

Place your fingertips on the floor to the right.
▸ Inhale, bend your right knee further and at the
same time lift your left leg so it is in line with your
body. Exhale, flex the left foot and keep both legs
straight. Release to the last position on page 77.
Repeat on the other side. ▸ Kneel on the right knee
and take your left leg to the side. Take your right
arm up and place your left hand on your left knee.
▸ Inhale, stretch to the left and slide your hand to

your ankle. Exhale then, breathing deeply, hold for
7–10 seconds. Repeat on the other side. ▸ Sit on the
floor, bend your left knee and place your right foot
flat on the floor so your knee is up. Place both palms
on the floor to the left. Inhale, bend your left elbow
and lift your right leg up in a 90-degree angle to the
floor. Clasp the two first fingers around the big toe
and flex the thumb. Exhale, breathe normally and
hold for 7 to 10 seconds. Repeat on the other side.

Day eight
BALANCE

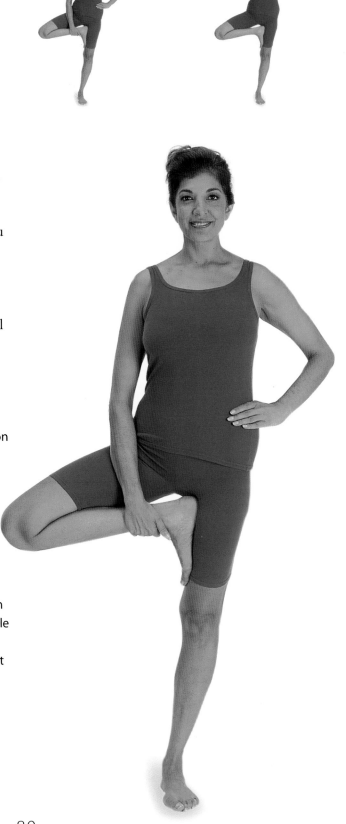

Yoga exercises unite mind and body and these balancing exercises will teach you how to focus your mind. In the beginning they may seem difficult, but with practice you will be surprised at how well you do; when your mind and body are in perfect harmony you will be absolutely still when you are holding a pose. The more you train your mind the longer you will be able to maintain the position. Some days you will feel off-balance when you wake up, and this is the right moment to bring yourself back to your center. When you are in perfect balance you will know it because your body will feel weightless and your mind will have an inner calm.

Stand tall, feet together and left hand on your waist. Lift your right leg and place your right foot on the inside of your left thigh. Focus your attention on one spot in front of you, grip the floor with your toes and lift the muscle above the kneecap of the standing leg to help you balance. Breathe normally. ▶ When you are absolutely still, place your palms in a prayer position. Hold for as long as you can. ▶ If possible, take your right leg into a half lotus position, the heel of your right foot close to your hipbone. Push your right knee back so your hips are square. Inhale and stretch your arms over your head, palms together. Exhale, breathe normally, and hold for at least 5 seconds. Inhale, exhale, and stretch to the right, keeping both hips square. Breathe normally and hold for 3 seconds. Inhale and return to the center. Exhale, and stretch over to the left. Return to the center. Repeat on the other side. ▶

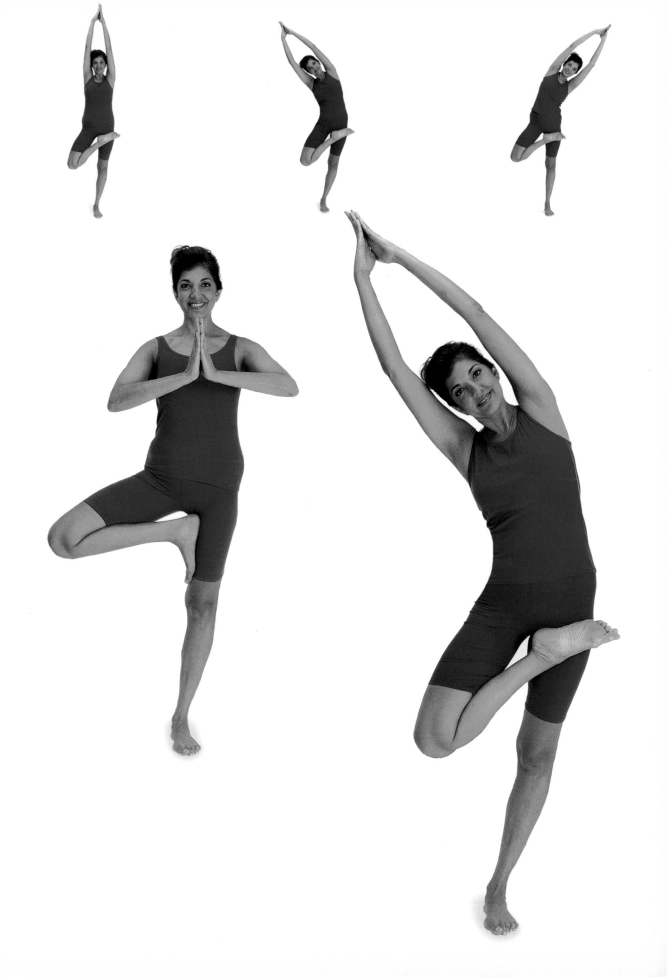

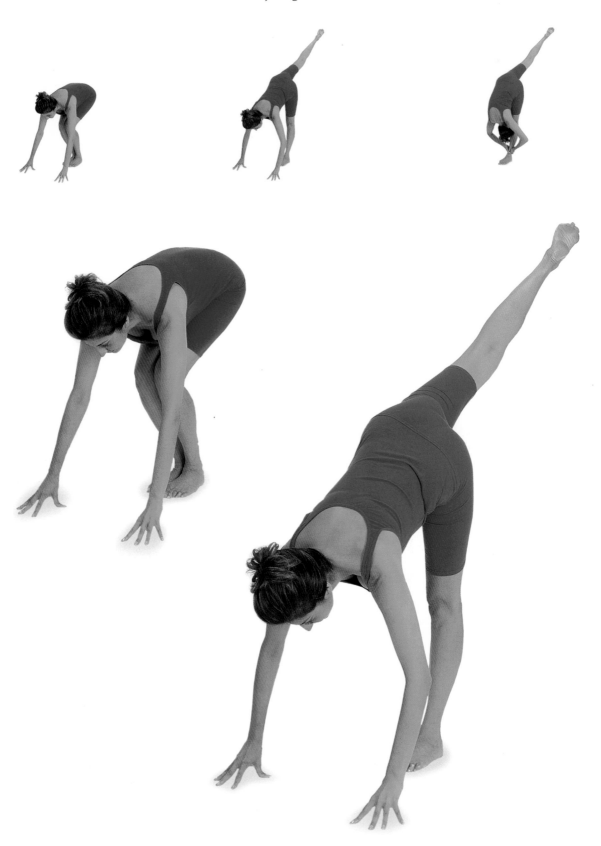

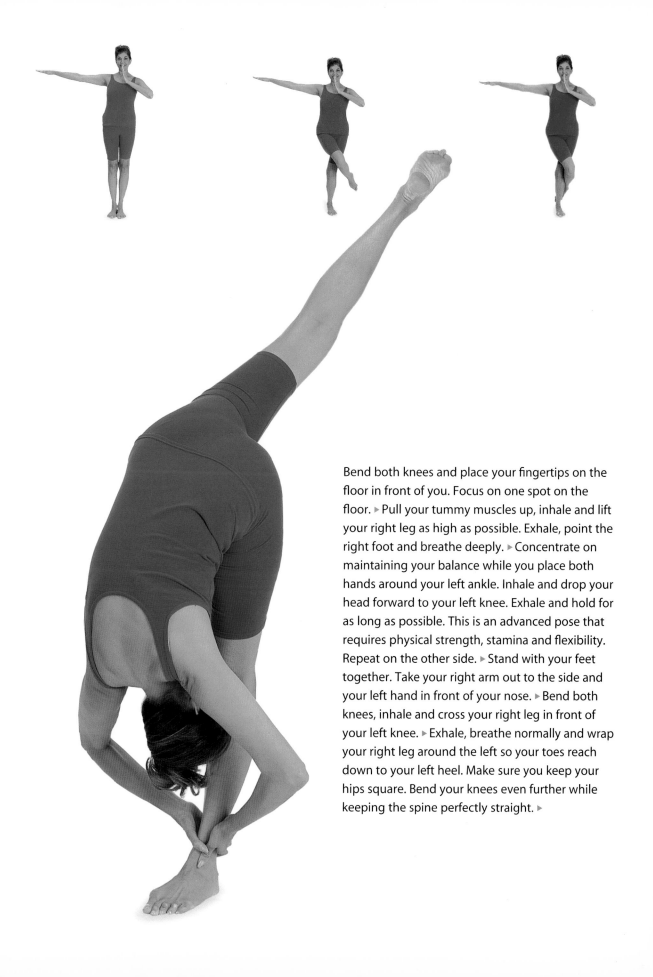

Bend both knees and place your fingertips on the floor in front of you. Focus on one spot on the floor. ▸ Pull your tummy muscles up, inhale and lift your right leg as high as possible. Exhale, point the right foot and breathe deeply. ▸ Concentrate on maintaining your balance while you place both hands around your left ankle. Inhale and drop your head forward to your left knee. Exhale and hold for as long as possible. This is an advanced pose that requires physical strength, stamina and flexibility. Repeat on the other side. ▸ Stand with your feet together. Take your right arm out to the side and your left hand in front of your nose. ▸ Bend both knees, inhale and cross your right leg in front of your left knee. ▸ Exhale, breathe normally and wrap your right leg around the left so your toes reach down to your left heel. Make sure you keep your hips square. Bend your knees even further while keeping the spine perfectly straight. ▸

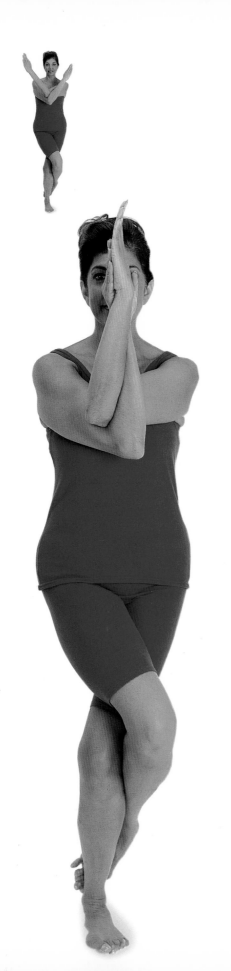

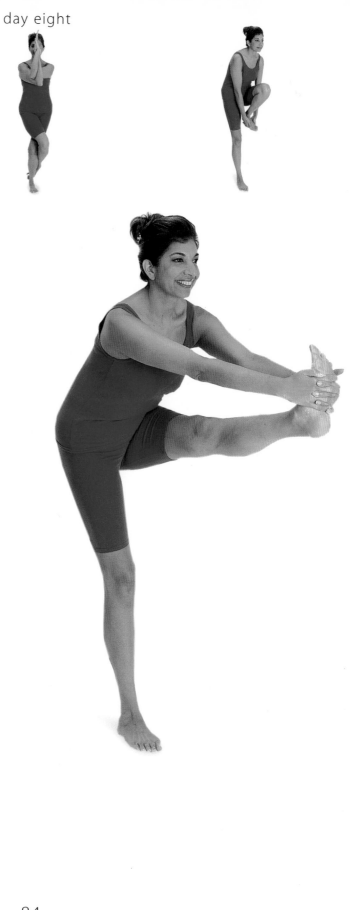

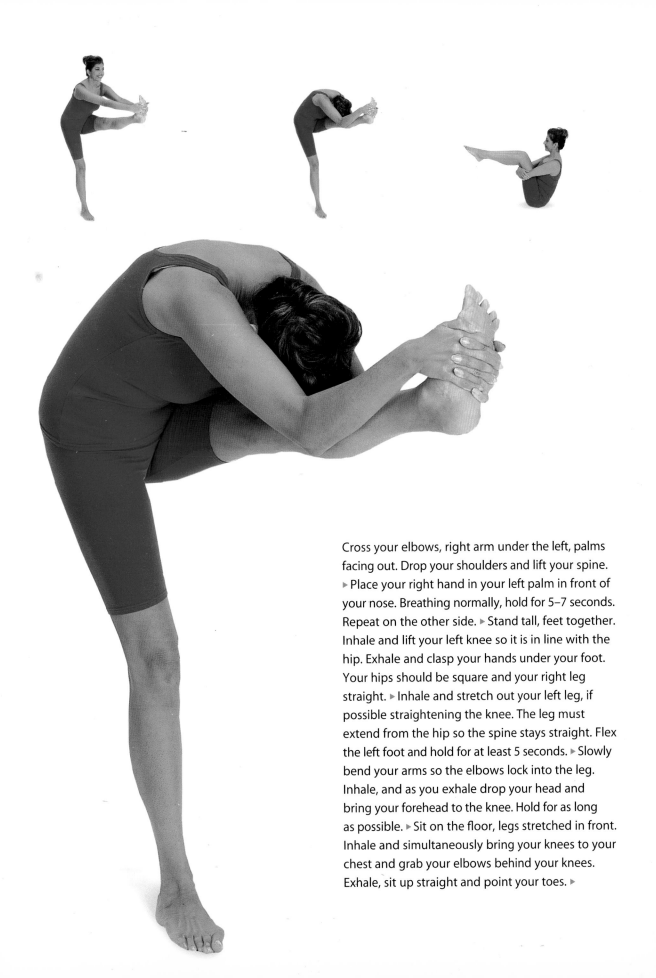

Cross your elbows, right arm under the left, palms facing out. Drop your shoulders and lift your spine. ▶ Place your right hand in your left palm in front of your nose. Breathing normally, hold for 5–7 seconds. Repeat on the other side. ▶ Stand tall, feet together. Inhale and lift your left knee so it is in line with the hip. Exhale and clasp your hands under your foot. Your hips should be square and your right leg straight. ▶ Inhale and stretch out your left leg, if possible straightening the knee. The leg must extend from the hip so the spine stays straight. Flex the left foot and hold for at least 5 seconds. ▶ Slowly bend your arms so the elbows lock into the leg. Inhale, and as you exhale drop your head and bring your forehead to the knee. Hold for as long as possible. ▶ Sit on the floor, legs stretched in front. Inhale and simultaneously bring your knees to your chest and grab your elbows behind your knees. Exhale, sit up straight and point your toes. ▶

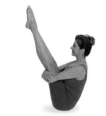

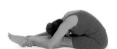

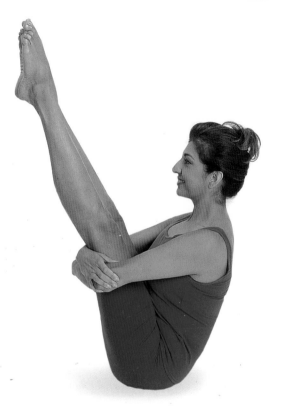

Breathing normally, straighten both legs so you are balancing on your buttock muscles. If you curve your spine you will roll backwards, so remember to tighten your tummy muscles and continue to sit upright. ▸ Release and bring both feet down to the floor. ▸ Inhale and as you exhale relax your legs forward and drop your head down to your knees. Breathe deeply and evenly and hold for 10 seconds. ▸ Uncurl your spine and sit up tall. Balance on your toes. Place your fingertips on the floor and cross your right leg over your left knee. Lean your body forward and place your right foot on the floor. ▸ Inhale, sit up tall and lift your right foot off the floor. Keep your fingertips down to help you balance. ▸ When you feel steady, bring your palms to your chest and balance on the ball of your left foot. Even if you hold this pose for just an instant you will feel elated. Repeat on the other side.

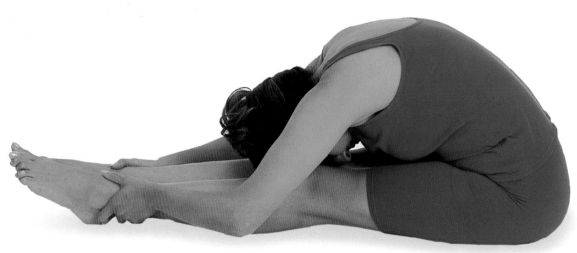

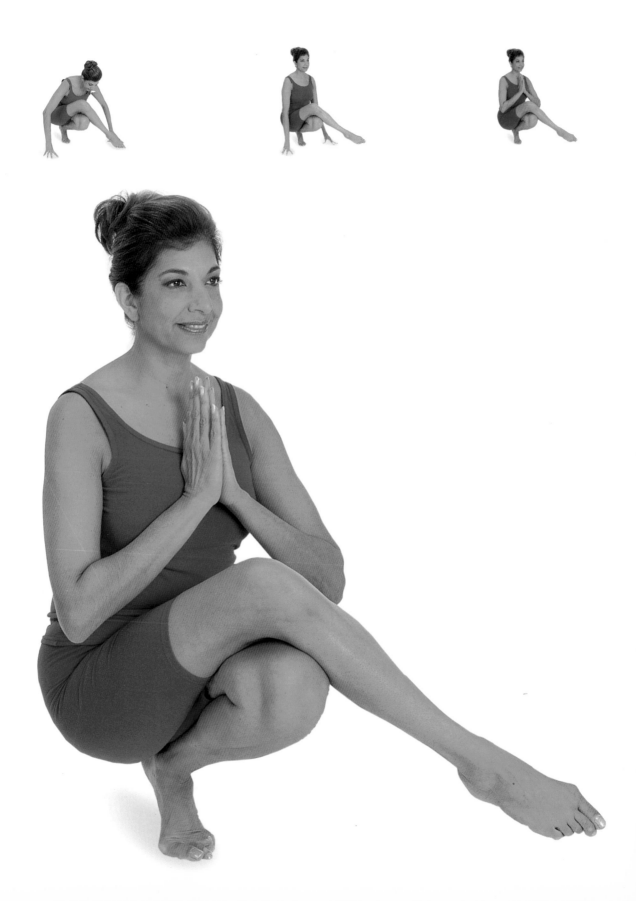

Day nine
REJUVENATION

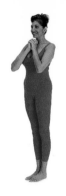 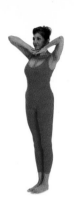

People who practise yoga always look younger than their years; their skin is clear, their eyes are bright and they seem to glow with well-being. The difference between yoga and other forms of exercise lies in the breathing techniques. *Pranayama*, or the science of breath, is the most important aspect of yoga philosophy. In this series of exercises, concentrate on breathing deeply and evenly throughout, taking slow and deliberate breaths. When you inhale, fill your lungs completely from the diaphragm. Keep your shoulders down and don't raise your chest. The movement should be concentrated only on the lower abdomen. As you exhale let the breath out slowly as you continue with the movement.

In this breathing exercise it is important to fill the lungs to their full capacity. This strengthens the respiratory wall and increases the fresh oxygen to the entire system. Keep the breath deep and even and let each movement flow from one to another. This breathing technique can be practised on its own or used as a warm-up to any of the exercise routines. ▸ Stand tall with your feet together. Interlace your fingers and place your hands under your chin. ▸ Inhale deeply and lift your elbows up as high as possible while keeping your head and chin level. ▸ Drop your head back, keeping your elbows up. ▸ Exhale through the mouth, blowing the air out slowly and evenly as you bring your elbows together. ▸ Inhale deeply, lift the elbows up in line with your shoulders and repeat the entire breathing exercise 7 times. Deepen the inhalation and exhalation as you continue this rejuvenating breathing technique. ▸

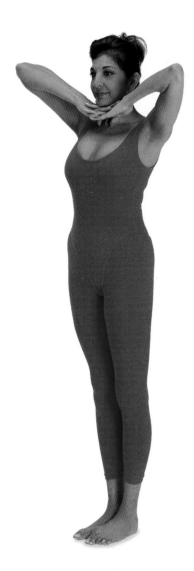

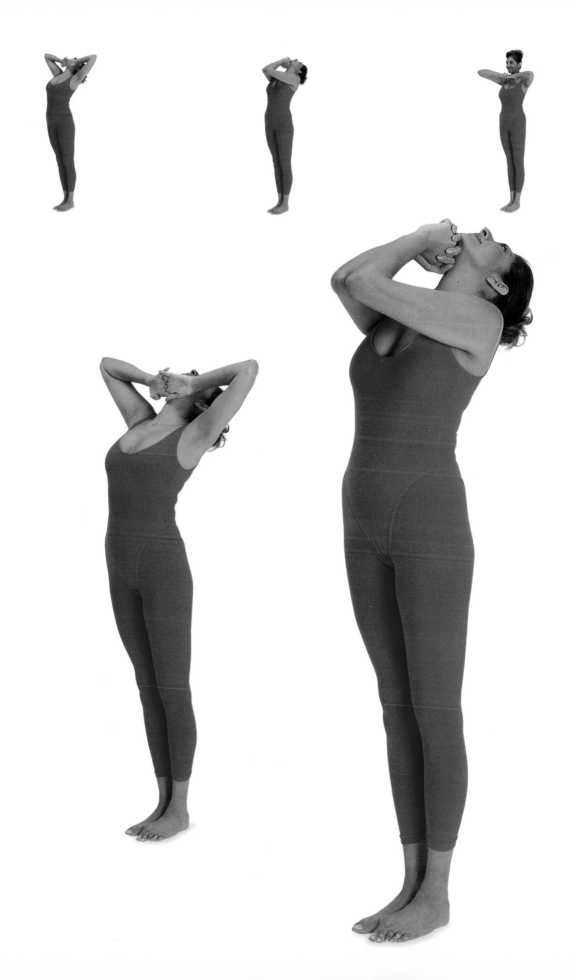

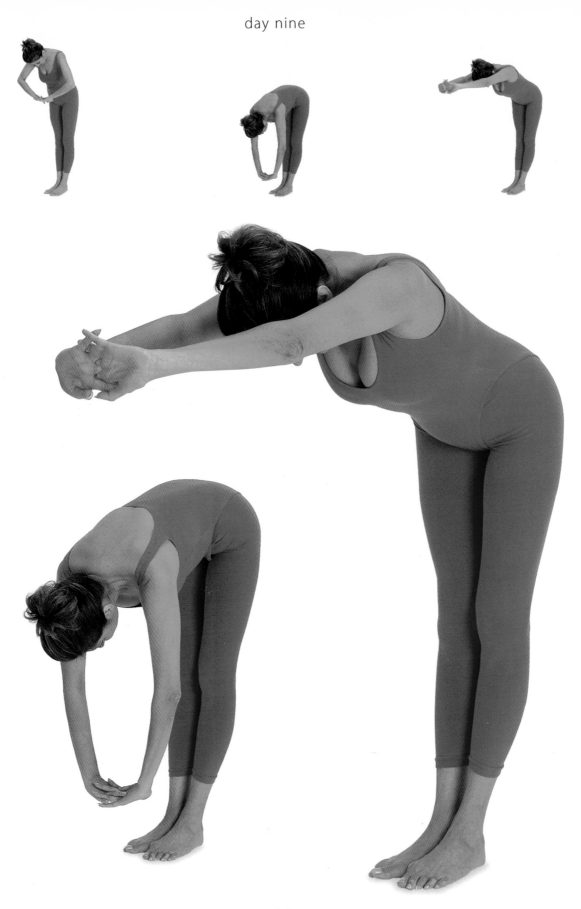

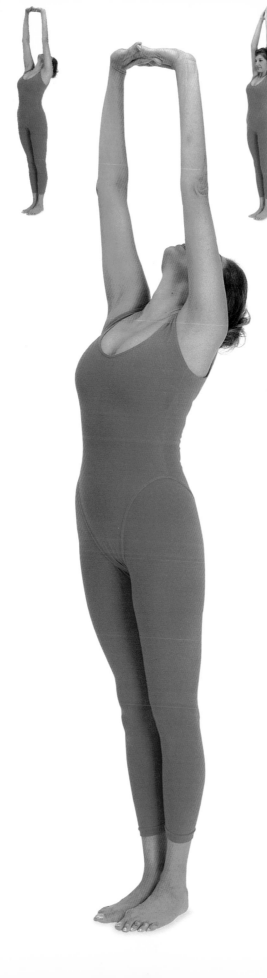
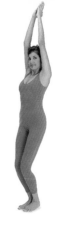

Inhale deeply and as you exhale slowly curve your spine, bend your elbows and drop your head forward, looking down to your fingertips. ▸ With a flowing movement, stretch your spine down and straighten your arms. Face your palms down towards your feet and let the natural weight of your body extend your spine further down. ▸ Inhale deeply and sweep your arms forward in a circular motion. Keep your head between your arms as you take your arms up over your head. ▸ Drop your head back and look up to your fingertips. Breathe deeply and evenly. Hold for 5 seconds. ▸ Straighten your head, bring your palms together and continue to stretch your arms up. Make sure your shoulders are down and your head is locked between your elbows. ▸ Keeping your spine straight, bend your knees, keeping your toes and heels firmly on the floor. Breathing deeply, hold for 5 seconds. ▸

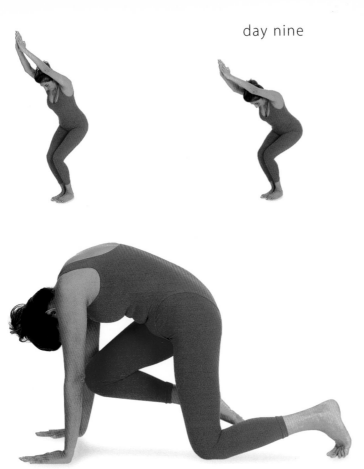

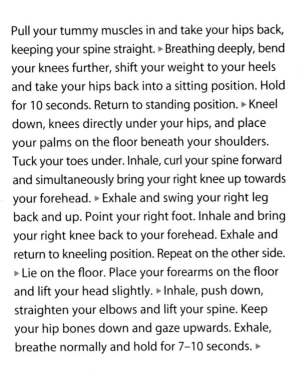

Pull your tummy muscles in and take your hips back, keeping your spine straight. ▸ Breathing deeply, bend your knees further, shift your weight to your heels and take your hips back into a sitting position. Hold for 10 seconds. Return to standing position. ▸ Kneel down, knees directly under your hips, and place your palms on the floor beneath your shoulders. Tuck your toes under. Inhale, curl your spine forward and simultaneously bring your right knee up towards your forehead. ▸ Exhale and swing your right leg back and up. Point your right foot. Inhale and bring your right knee back to your forehead. Exhale and return to kneeling position. Repeat on the other side. ▸ Lie on the floor. Place your forearms on the floor and lift your head slightly. ▸ Inhale, push down, straighten your elbows and lift your spine. Keep your hip bones down and gaze upwards. Exhale, breathe normally and hold for 7–10 seconds. ▸

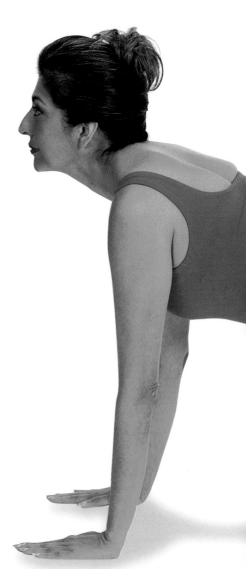

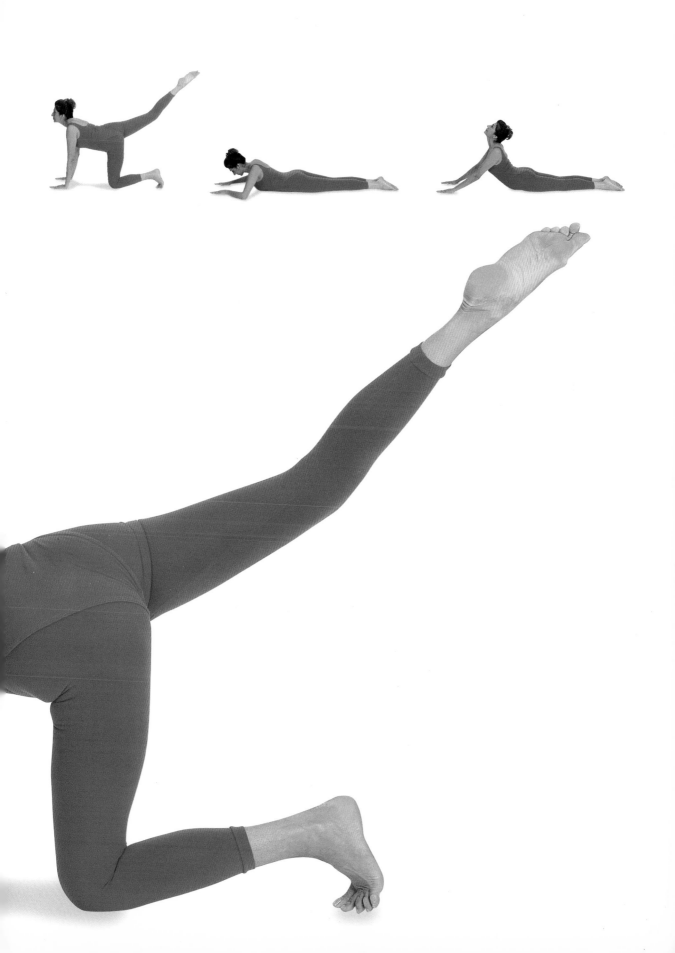

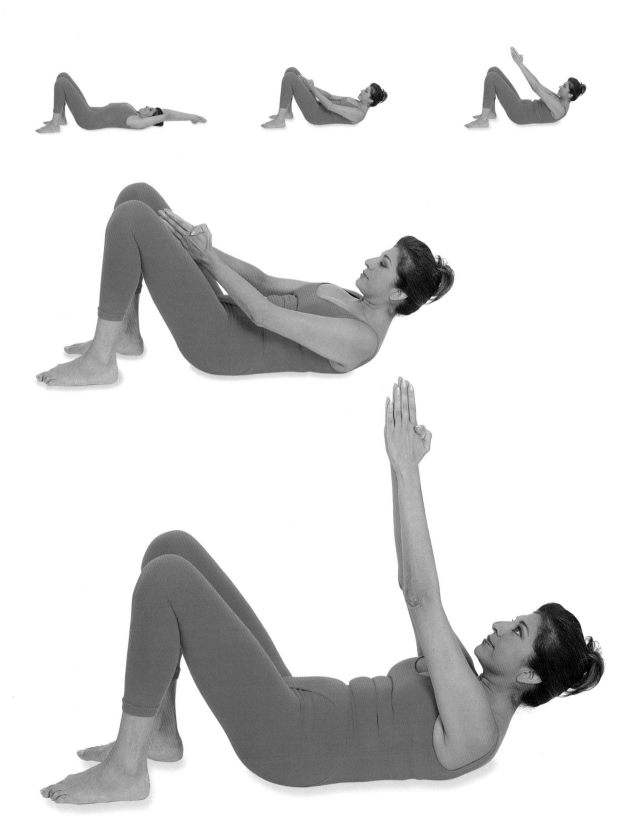

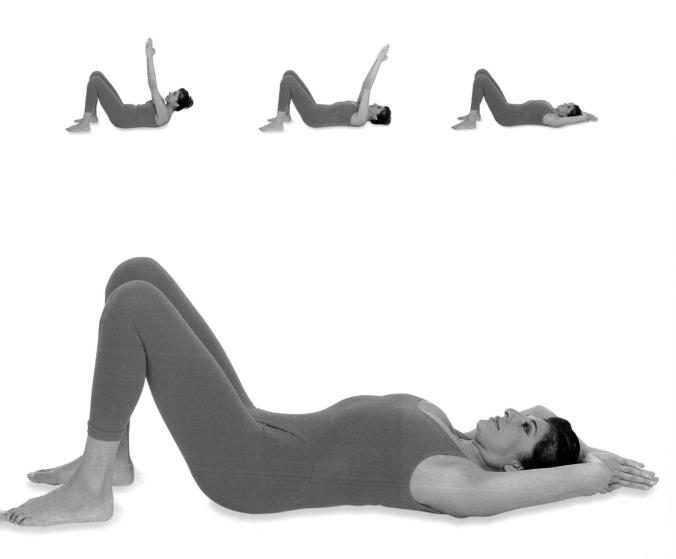

Lie flat on the floor. Bring your knees up directly in line with your hips. Put your palms together and stretch your arms over your head. ▸ Inhale and as you exhale tighten your tummy muscles and bring your hands over your head to your knees, slowly lifting your head and shoulders off the floor. ▸ Sitting up further, inhale and raise your arms above your knees. ▸ Exhale, lower your back halfway down to the floor and bring your arms up in a straight line to your shoulders. ▸ Inhale and take your arms over your head as you slowly lower your spine to the floor. Exhale and lower your arms to the floor. ▸ Inhale, bend your elbows and bring your hands over the top of your head, palms together. Repeat the entire series 5 times. Keep the breathing pattern fluid as you move from one position to the next. Hold your breath for 2 seconds in each position to gain breath control.

Day ten
CALMING THE NERVOUS SYSTEM

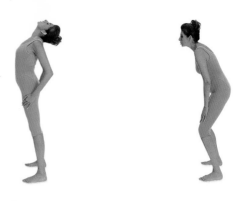

Deep breathing acts as a tranquillizer to the nervous system, and when it is combined with forward bends the blood supply rushes to the head, calming and soothing the brain. As you begin this section keep in mind that you wish to release all the longstanding tension in your mind and body. Try to hold the positions for as long as possible to allow deep relaxation of every nerve, and as you breathe through the exercises let the rhythm of the breath release all mental, emotional and physical ailments. This relaxation technique can be used to lead you to a peaceful slumber or, if you need to pep yourself up in the middle of the day, practise it for 15 minutes and you will feel as refreshed as if you have just woken up from a good night's sleep.

Stand tall, your feet 30–60 cm (1–2 ft) apart and your arms to the side. As you inhale as deeply as possible, drop your head back and bend your elbows. ▸ Open your mouth and release the breath slowly, making a 'swoosh' sound, at the same time placing your hands to your thighs and beginning to drop your head forward until you curve your spine down and you are out of breath. ▸ When all the breath is out of your body move your hands to face one another. ▸ Contract your tummy muscles so they move under the ribcage. Push the tummy muscles in and out one more time without inhaling. Inhale through your nose and stand up tall. Repeat. ▸ Kneel on the floor, knees hip width apart, and place your hands in line with your shoulders. Repeat the breathing exercise in this position. ▸

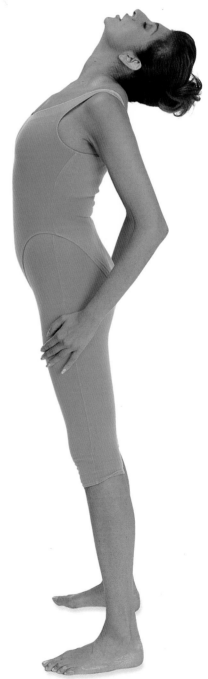

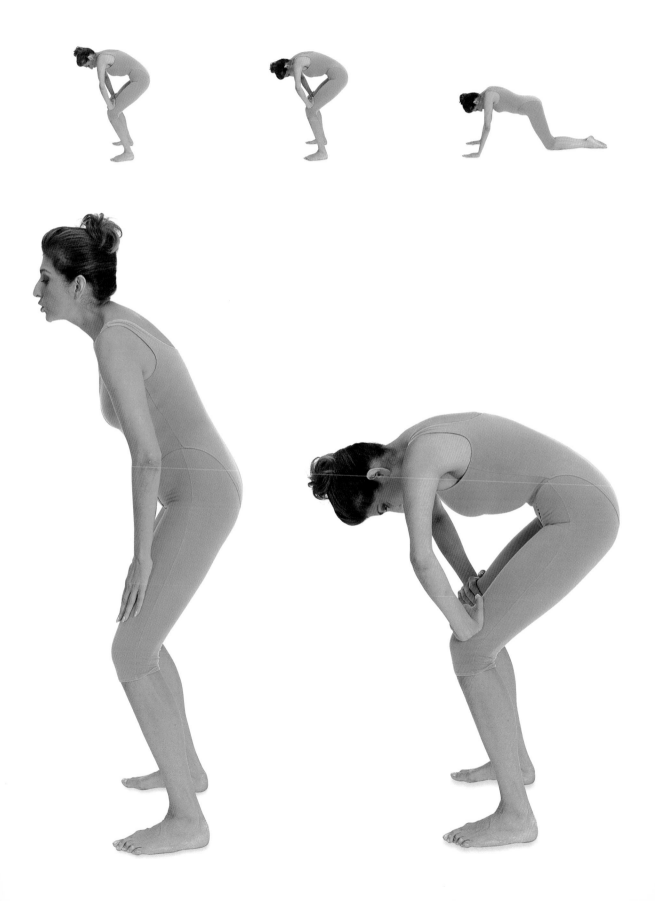

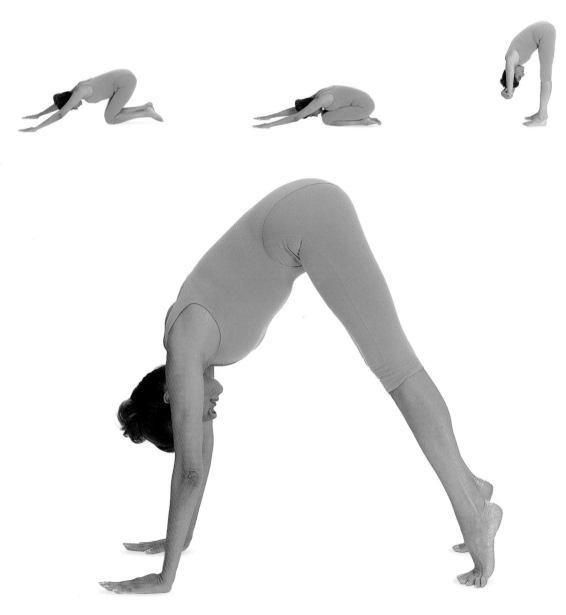

Inhale and, without moving your hands, slowly stretch your spine. Exhale and hold for 5 seconds, breathing deeply. ▸ Inhale and rest your hips back on your heels. Exhale and relax your forehead down to the floor. Breathing normally, hold for 7–10 seconds. ▸ Stand tall, feet 30 cm (1 ft) apart, holding your elbows. Stretching forward from the tailbone, relax your entire spine. ▸ Inhale, tighten your tummy muscles and take your arms over your head. Exhale, breathe deeply and hold for 7–10 seconds. Place your palms on the floor and walk your hands forward. Balance on your toes. ▸ Inhale, pull up your tummy muscles and lower your heels to the floor. Exhale, breathe deeply and hold for 7–10 seconds. ▸Inhale and lift your right leg up behind you in a diagonal line, foot flexed. Exhale, breathe deeply and hold for 5 seconds. Slowly lower your leg. Repeat on the other side. ▸

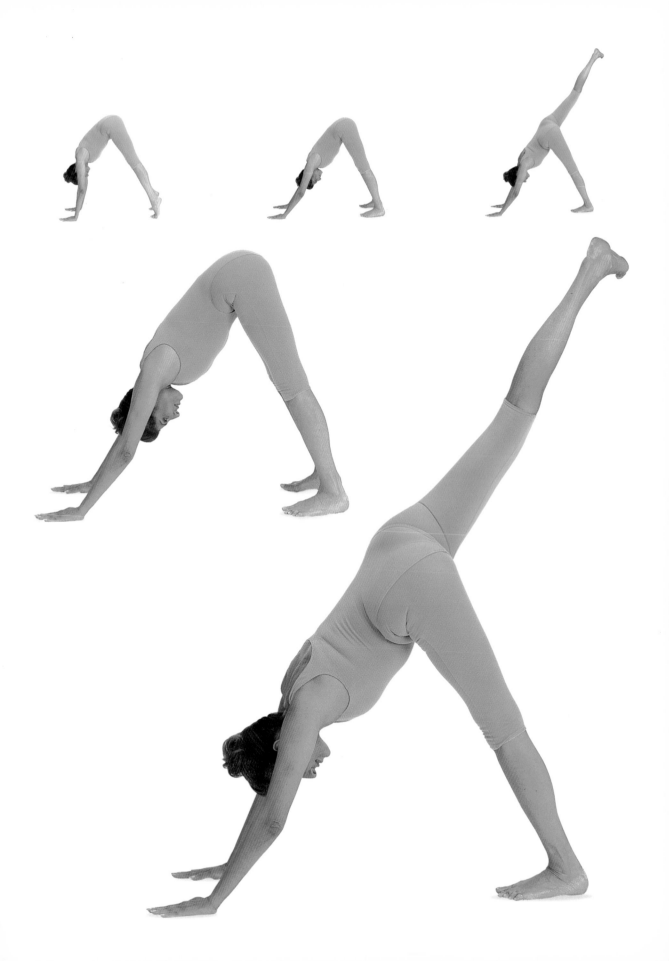

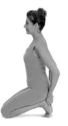

Sit down on your heels. Tuck your toes under and hold on to your heels. ▶ Place your forehead down to the floor close to your knees. ▶ Inhale, straighten your arms and roll forward on to the top of your head. Exhale, breathe normally and hold for 7–10 seconds. While you are in this position you will feel the blood rush to your head. This sensation can feel uncomfortable at first but with continued practice it becomes pleasant. ▶ Sit down with your legs outstretched in front of you. Inhale and raise your arms out to the side in line with your shoulders. ▶ Exhale, inhale, point your toes and raise your arms up over your head with your palms facing each other. Look up towards your hands and hold for 2 seconds. ▶ Exhale and stretch forward from the tailbone. Keep your head in line with your arms and face your hands down towards your feet. Breathe deeply as you slowly stretch forward towards your legs. ▶

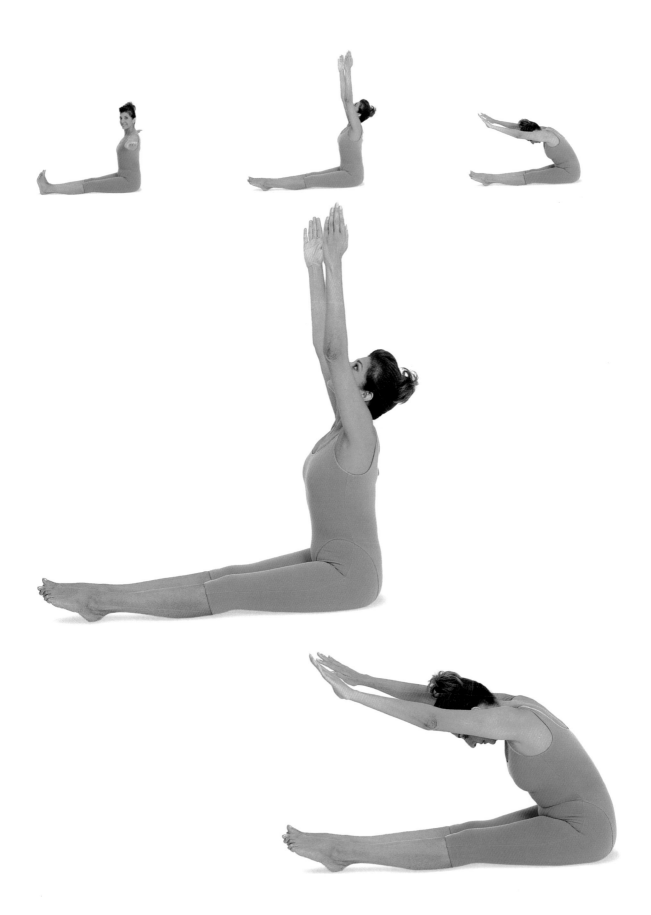

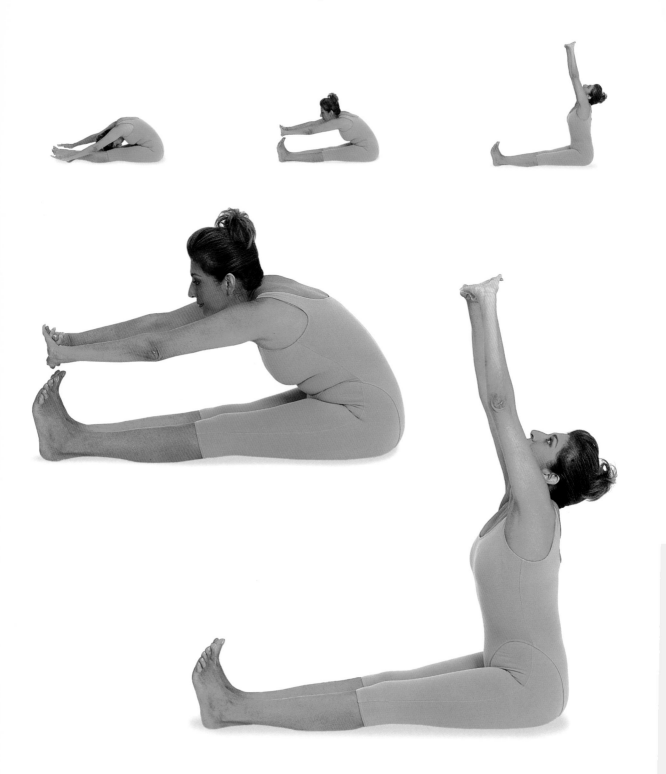
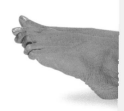

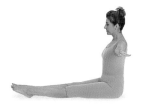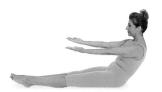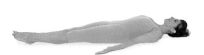

Breathing deeply and evenly, relax your spine all the way down so your forehead touches your knees. If you are unable to stretch all the way down do not force your body – let your natural weight combined with deep breathing relax your spine. Hold for 7–10 seconds. ▸ Flex your feet and interlace your fingers, palms facing out. ▸ Inhale and stretch your arms forward and over your head. Straighten your spine and look up towards your hands. Exhale, breathe

normally and hold for 5 seconds. ▸ Exhale, point your toes and release your arms to your sides. Drop your shoulders, extend your arms and keep your fingers together and palms facing down. ▸ Concentrating on your tummy muscles, inhale, turn your palms upwards and slowly lower your spine to the floor. ▸ Exhale and breathe deeply and evenly as you relax every muscle. If you remain in this relaxation pose for 15 minutes you will feel totally refreshed.

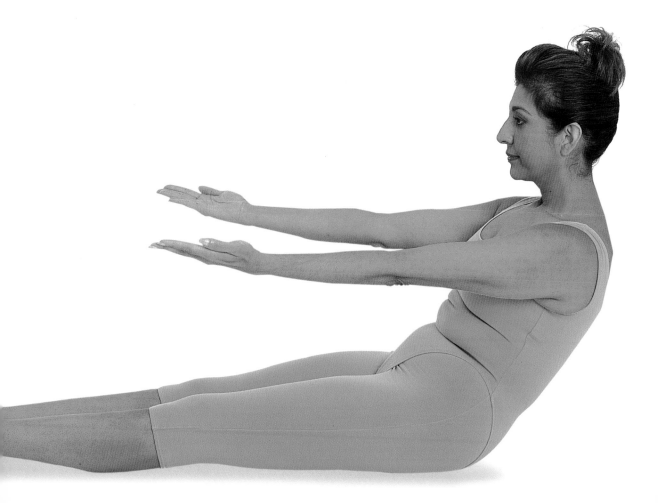

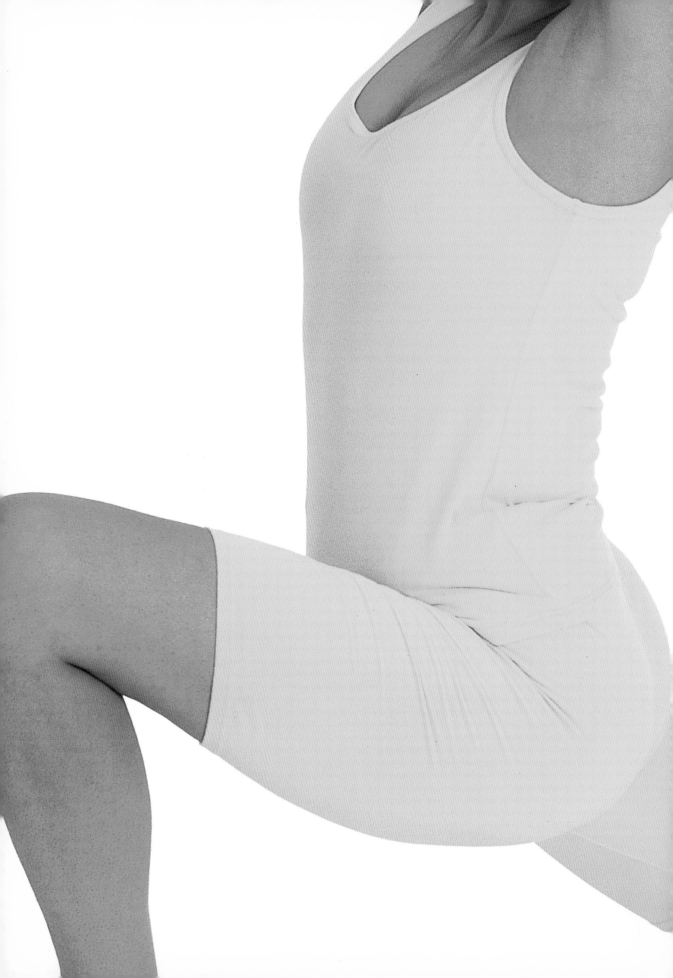

MAINTENANCE

The Round-the-Body routine is a ten minute exercise plan that tones and lifts the specific muscle groups that show the first signs of ageing. If your body is losing its elasticity and your muscles are beginning to sag it is important to address the problem before it becomes severe – but it is better still to keep yourself in shape and use this plan as a preventive measure. These exercises are designed to lift the entire body to restore youthfulness and suppleness; they will tone the ankles, calves, kneecaps and upper thighs, flatten the tummy, lift the buttocks and reduce the hips and waist. Stretching upwards will tighten the muscles around the ribcage and in the upper arms and lift the breasts, while the twisting and turning of the body will increase the circulation to the face, which will reduce fine lines and wrinkles. It is a dynamic fitness routine that can be done on its own or for increased benefit can be combined with any Day plan or with the Warm-up, depending on how much time you have or what specific areas you need to work on. It can also be a preface to the Remedial exercises which appear in the latter half of this section. Because the Remedial section targets specific problem areas, you will notice the results in a surprisingly short time. Doctors now agree that there is a direct link between the emotional balance of a person and their susceptibility to certain illnesses – people suffering from stomach cramps, for example, are often emotionally upset. They commonly take medication to relieve their pain, but yoga will relax the stomach cramps immediately because it teaches you to breathe through the pain in order to release it. Because it tones, reoxygenates and rejuvenates the entire body, it can alleviate a whole range of common problems, both physical and mental.

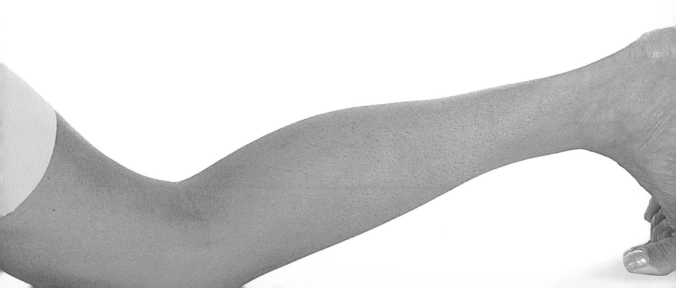

Round-the-Body
SALUTE TO THE SUN

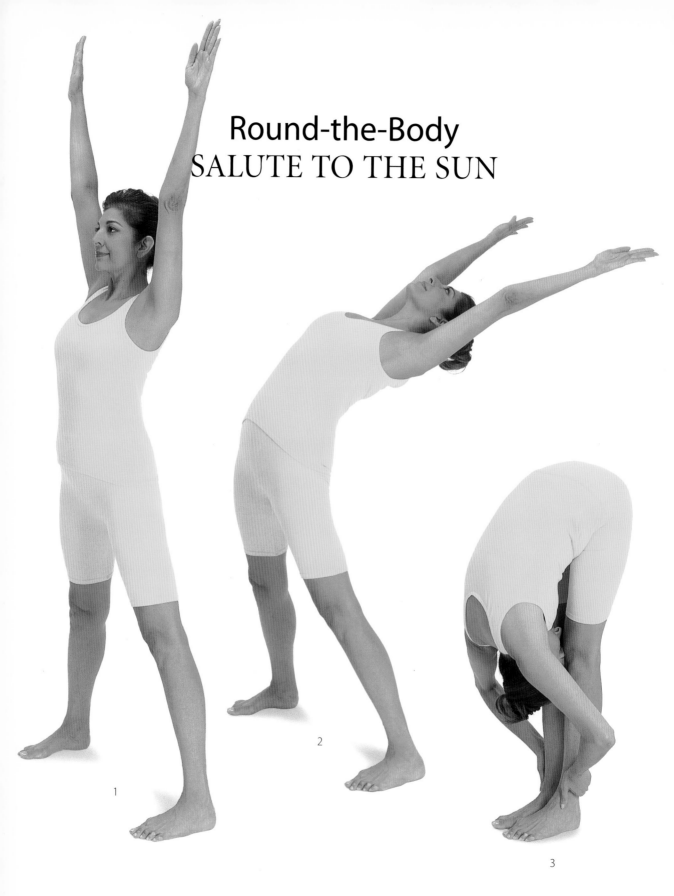

1

2

3

Stand tall, feet together and arms at the side. Take your right foot 60 cm (2 ft) to the right. Raise both arms over your head, palms facing forward. Keep your shoulders down. ▸ Inhale deeply and bend your body back as far as possible. Keep your arms in line with your head and your palms upwards. ▸ Exhale, bring your right foot to your left and take your arms up to the starting position. Continuing to exhale, stretch your arms forward and relax your spine. Hold your ankles and stretch your forehead down to your knees. ▸ Bend your left knee, place your fingertips on the floor and take your right foot back as far as possible, toes tucked under. ▸ Inhale, drop your right knee to the floor, lift your spine and stretch your arms over your head. Cross your thumbs, place your palms together and straighten your elbows. Make sure you are balancing on the top of your right knee to avoid injury to the kneecap. Exhale, bring both feet together and repeat on the other side.

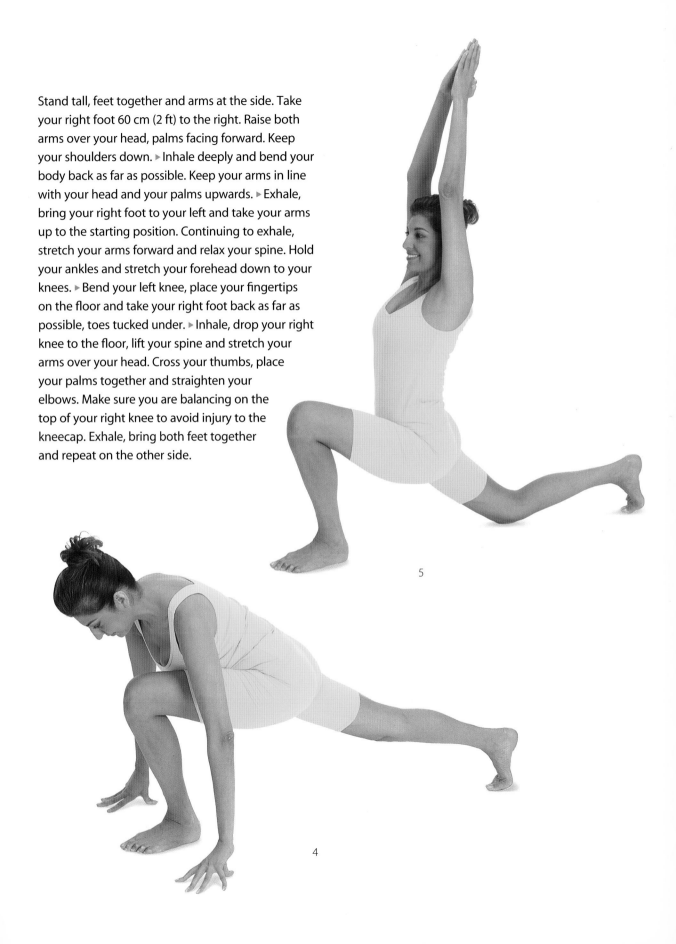

5

4

WARRIOR

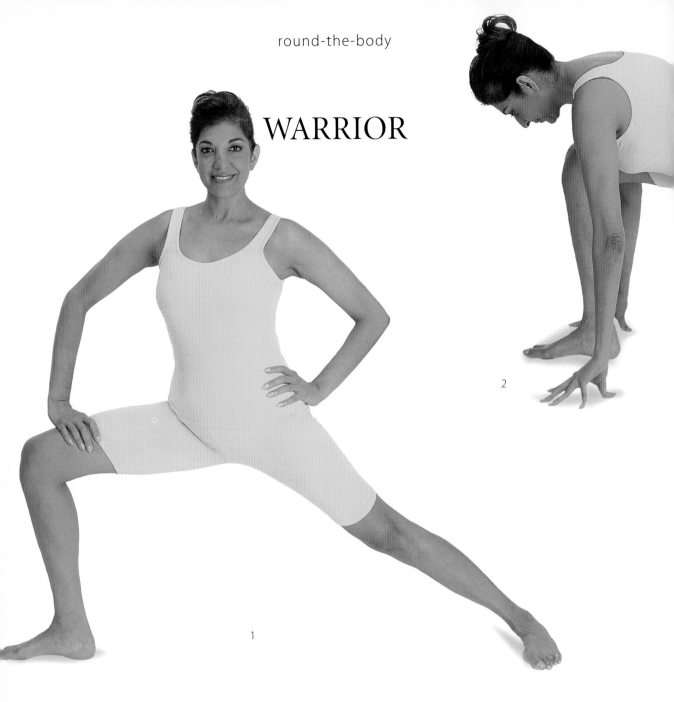

1

2

Stand with your feet 1–1.2 m (3–4 ft) apart, arms to the side. Turn your right foot to the right with your right heel in a direct line to the instep of your left foot. Bend your right knee in a 90-degree angle so the back of the knee is in line with the right heel. Take your right hand to your inner thigh and your left hand to your waist. Breathing normally, hold for 5–7 seconds. ▶ Turn your body to the right and place your fingertips on the floor. Turn your left foot so it is in line with your right heel. ▶ Bend your left arm and place your elbow on the outside of your right knee. Keep your fingers together and look down at your palm. ▶ Inhale, twist your spine to the right and look over your right shoulder. Take your right hand round to your left hip and your left hand to the floor beside your right leg. Exhale, breathe deeply and hold for 7–10 seconds. Release, stand tall and repeat on the other side.

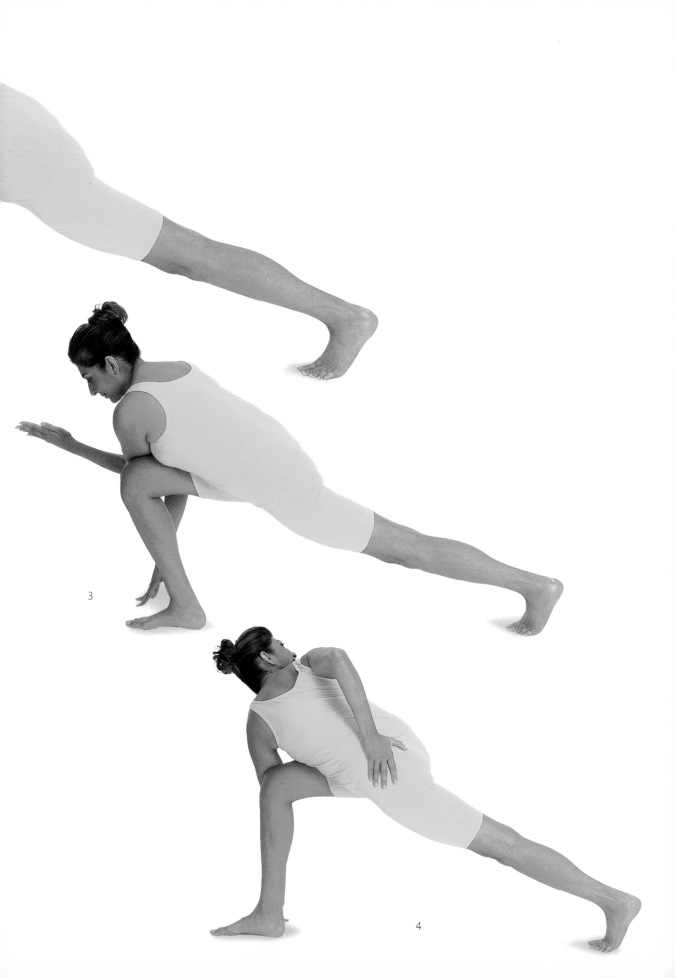

3

4

STOMACH STRETCHES

This series of movements will tighten and tone the lower abdominal muscles and flatten the tummy. Pay extra attention to the breathing pattern for the best results; breathing incorrectly may even build the muscles so your tummy actually appears larger. Lie flat on the floor with your arms to the side. Bring your left knee up and place your left foot flat on the floor. Point your right foot and take both arms over your head. Place your palms together and straighten your elbows. ▸ Inhale and lift your right leg up to a 90-degree angle. Exhale, breathe normally and hold for 5 seconds. ▸ Inhale and bring your palms in towards your head. Exhale, sit up and bring your arms down in front of your face above the chest. ▸ Inhale, straighten your arms, exhale, breathe normally and hold for 5 seconds. Inhale, slowly lower your back and take your arms over your head. Exhale and then repeat the exercise on the other side.

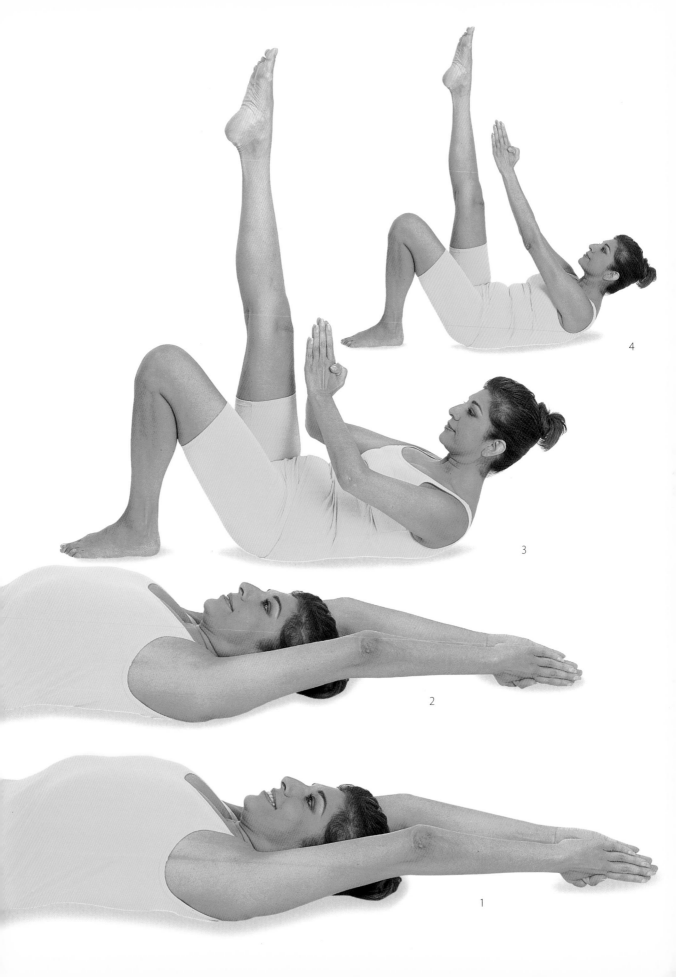

4

3

2

1

PUSH-UPS

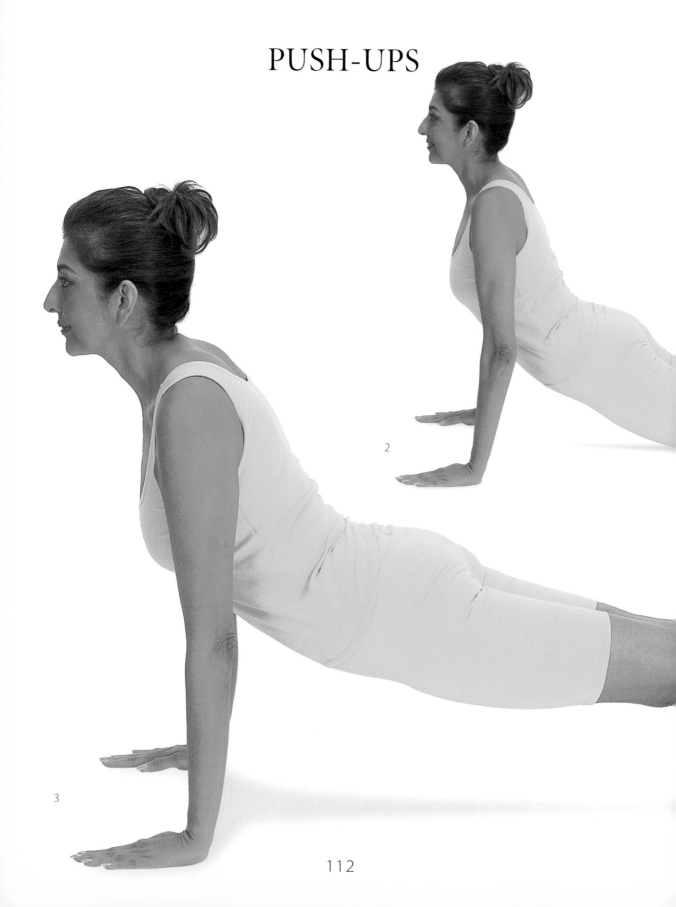

2

3

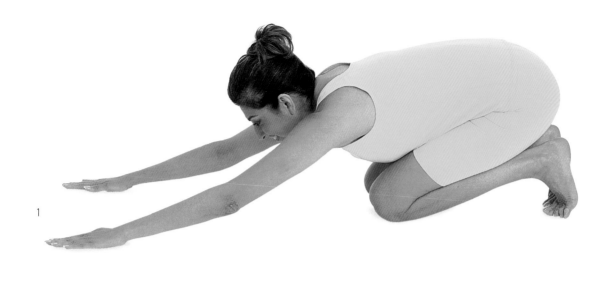

1

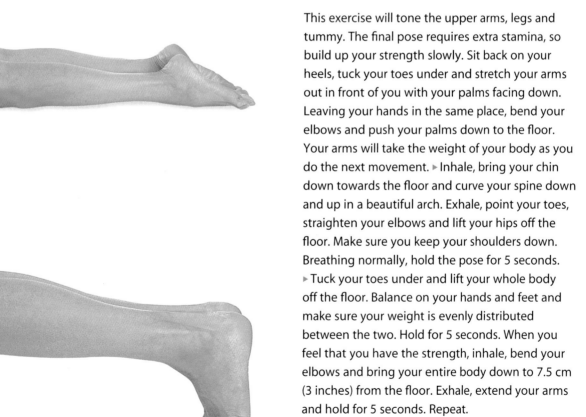

This exercise will tone the upper arms, legs and tummy. The final pose requires extra stamina, so build up your strength slowly. Sit back on your heels, tuck your toes under and stretch your arms out in front of you with your palms facing down. Leaving your hands in the same place, bend your elbows and push your palms down to the floor. Your arms will take the weight of your body as you do the next movement. ▸ Inhale, bring your chin down towards the floor and curve your spine down and up in a beautiful arch. Exhale, point your toes, straighten your elbows and lift your hips off the floor. Make sure you keep your shoulders down. Breathing normally, hold the pose for 5 seconds. ▸ Tuck your toes under and lift your whole body off the floor. Balance on your hands and feet and make sure your weight is evenly distributed between the two. Hold for 5 seconds. When you feel that you have the strength, inhale, bend your elbows and bring your entire body down to 7.5 cm (3 inches) from the floor. Exhale, extend your arms and hold for 5 seconds. Repeat.

TABLE TOP

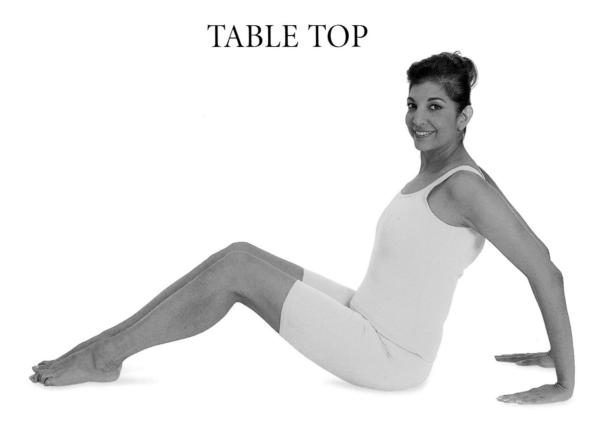

1

This exercise will tone every muscle in your body at once and requires flexibility, strength and stamina. It will help to focus your mind as well as giving you a feeling of inner balance and harmony. It is a challenging pose so it might take you some time and practice to master it. Sit down with your legs outstretched in front of you. Point your toes, leave your feet flat down and bring your knees slightly off the floor in line with your waist. Lean back and take your arms behind you so your hands are hip-width apart and your fingers are facing your body. ▸ Straighten your arms, tighten your tummy and buttock muscles, inhale and lift your whole body off the floor. ▸ Exhale, inhale and to increase the stretch contract your buttock muscles and lift your hips higher off the floor so your body is in a perfect diagonal line. Exhale and drop your head back. Breathe normally and hold this intense stretch for 5–7 seconds. To release, sit back down on the floor.

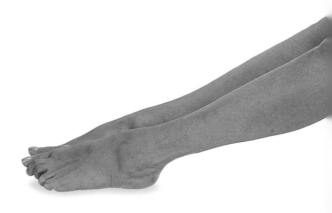

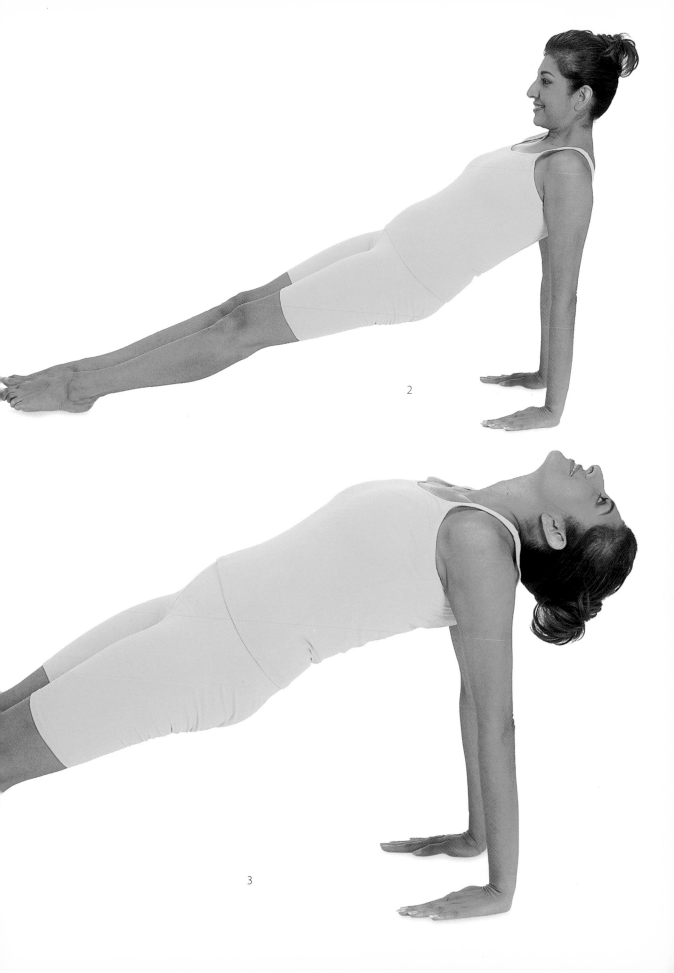

2

3

Remedial
ARTHRITIS

This is an excellent way to relieve stiffness in the joints, especially in the feet, hands, knees, hips and shoulders. In the beginning this exercise might feel uncomfortable but continued practice will alleviate the pain and increase circulation to the joints. Kneel up tall then tuck the toes under and sit back on to the heels. If you feel any pain release the toes and continue with the exercise. ▸ Place your hands behind you for support, fingers pointing away from you. Keep your arms and spine straight. Breathing normally, lift your hips up and push them forward as high as possible while balancing on your hands. Your weight should be evenly distributed between your arms and hips. ▸ Drop your head back, lifting your chin and hips up to create a circular pattern with your spine. Hold for at least 5 seconds and repeat. When you are able to hold this pose comfortably increase to 10 seconds.

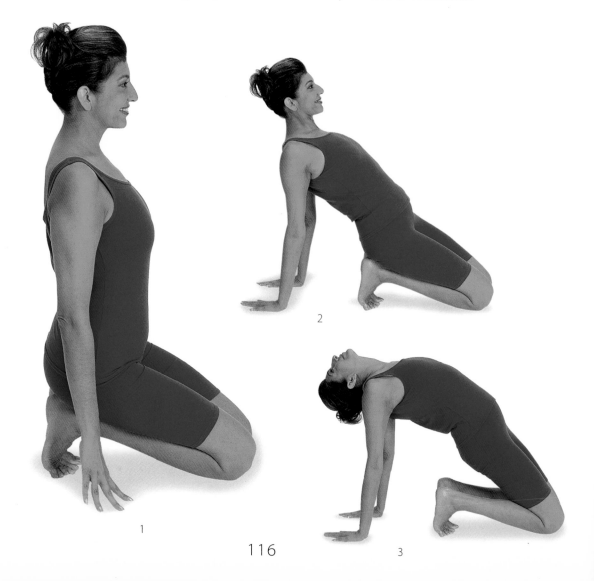

1

2

3

OSTEOPOROSIS

As you age it is vital to take extra calcium to stop the bones from becoming brittle. Equally important in preventing this condition from occurring is keeping a fresh blood supply to the hip area. This twist sends fresh oxygen and a purified blood supply to the hips and increases the circulation of the entire system. It alleviates painful conditions like sciatica as well as strengthening the hip joints. Stand tall with your feet 1–1.2 m (3–4 ft) apart. Turn your left foot to the left and make sure your left heel is in a direct line with the instep of your right foot. Take your arms out to the side in line with your shoulders. Bend your right elbow so it is in line with your left knee.

▸ Inhale, put your right hand on the floor, exhale, twist your spine and look up over your left shoulder. Breathe deeply and hold for 5–7 seconds. Keep your arms in a straight line. If you are unable to touch the floor with your hand hold any part of your left leg. Repeat on the other side.

2

1

IMMUNE SYSTEM

When the immune system is weak the body is vulnerable to all kinds of health problems. Stress weakens the immune system, but even though it is hard to eliminate stress from our daily lives we can learn to boost the immune system in order to prevent ailments from becoming chronic. Sit sideways on the floor, leaning on your right hip. Straighten your right leg and point your toe. Take your left knee up so your left foot is flat on the floor behind the right knee. Place your right palm on the floor about 30 cm (1 ft) from your right hip. Place your left hand near the upper thigh of your right leg. ▸ Inhale and push yourself up, balancing on your right hand and right foot. Exhale, keeping the legs parallel and your right arm fully extended. Your left arm should be pointed straight up in the air in line with your right arm. Breathe deeply and hold for as long as you can. Repeat on the other side.

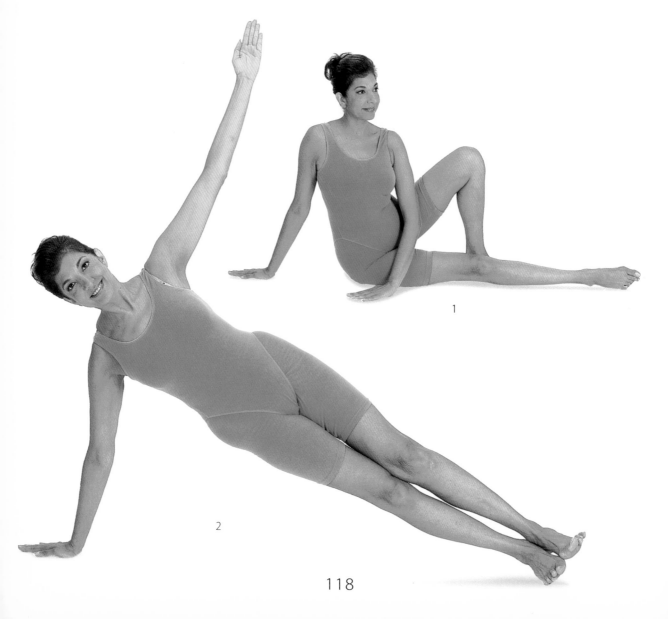

1

2

INSOMNIA

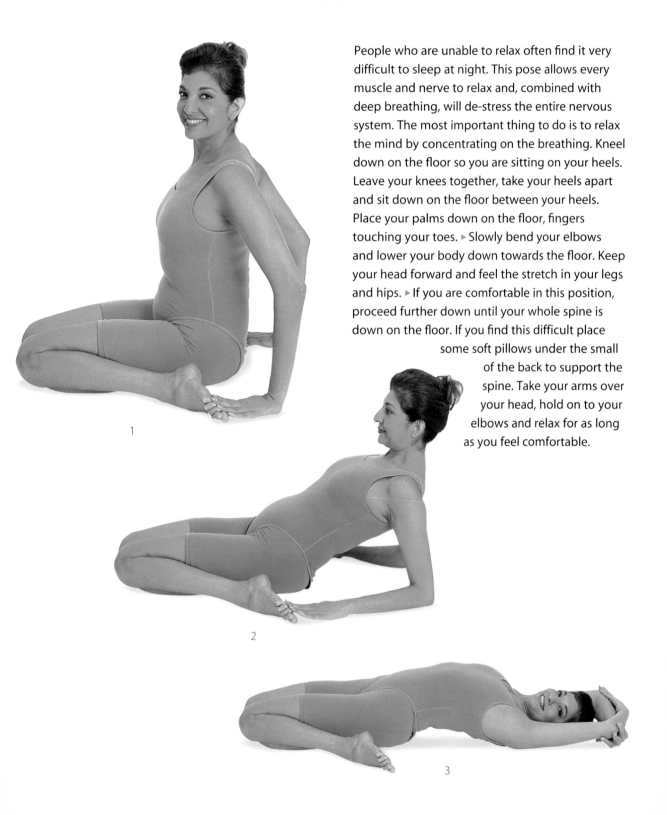

People who are unable to relax often find it very difficult to sleep at night. This pose allows every muscle and nerve to relax and, combined with deep breathing, will de-stress the entire nervous system. The most important thing to do is to relax the mind by concentrating on the breathing. Kneel down on the floor so you are sitting on your heels. Leave your knees together, take your heels apart and sit down on the floor between your heels. Place your palms down on the floor, fingers touching your toes. ▶ Slowly bend your elbows and lower your body down towards the floor. Keep your head forward and feel the stretch in your legs and hips. ▶ If you are comfortable in this position, proceed further down until your whole spine is down on the floor. If you find this difficult place some soft pillows under the small of the back to support the spine. Take your arms over your head, hold on to your elbows and relax for as long as you feel comfortable.

1

2

3

DEPRESSION

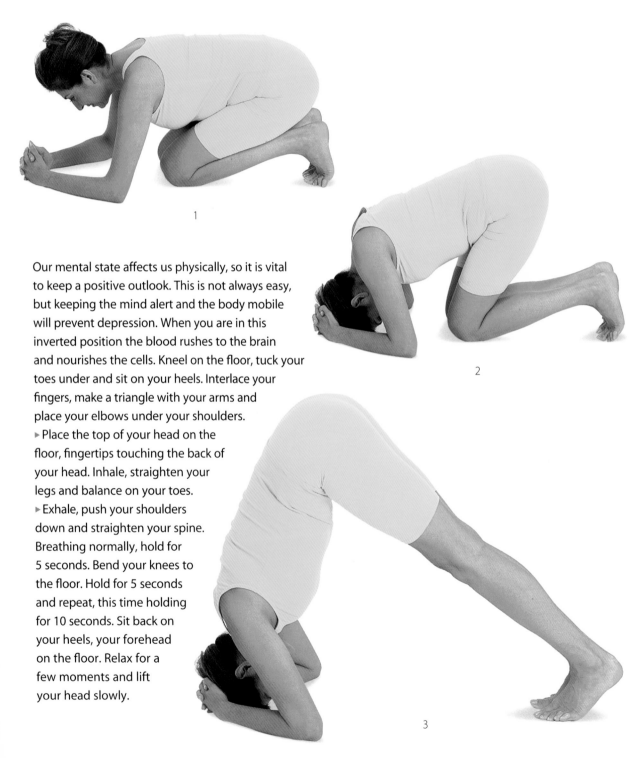

1

Our mental state affects us physically, so it is vital to keep a positive outlook. This is not always easy, but keeping the mind alert and the body mobile will prevent depression. When you are in this inverted position the blood rushes to the brain and nourishes the cells. Kneel on the floor, tuck your toes under and sit on your heels. Interlace your fingers, make a triangle with your arms and place your elbows under your shoulders.

▶ Place the top of your head on the floor, fingertips touching the back of your head. Inhale, straighten your legs and balance on your toes.

▶ Exhale, push your shoulders down and straighten your spine. Breathing normally, hold for 5 seconds. Bend your knees to the floor. Hold for 5 seconds and repeat, this time holding for 10 seconds. Sit back on your heels, your forehead on the floor. Relax for a few moments and lift your head slowly.

2

3

EYE STRAIN

As people age the eye muscles become lax. These exercises are designed to strengthen the eye muscles so vision is improved. Sit up tall in a comfortable cross-legged position. Straighten your index finger and place it in front of your nose. Stretch your right arm out in front of you and stare at your finger for 5 seconds. ▸ Keeping your eyes focused on your finger, slowly bring it towards you until it touches the tip of your nose. Still keeping your eyes focused on your finger, stretch the arm out again. Rub your hands and place your palms over your eyes. ▸ Keeping your head straight, take your arm up to the right, eyes still focused on your finger. ▸ Then take your arm diagonally to the left. Repeat on the same side, then on other side. Rub your hands together and cup them over your eyes.

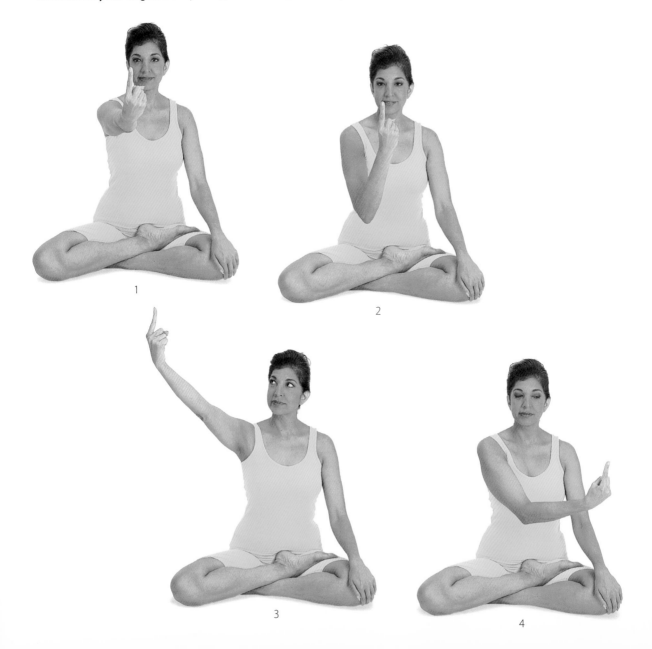

1

2

3

4

PELVIC FLOOR

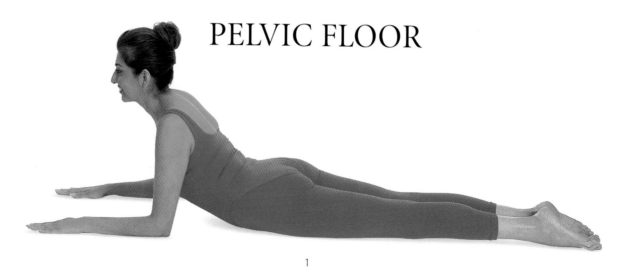

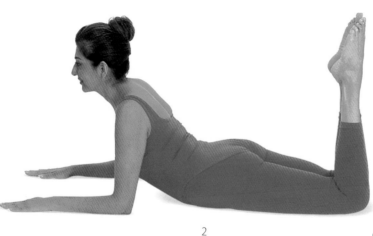

1

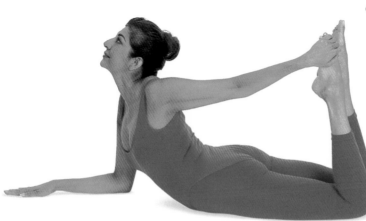

2

After childbirth and with advancing age, many women suffer from incontinence and other urinary disorders. The pelvic floor must be kept toned in order for the urinary system and sexual organs to function properly. As you do the following exercise, contract the pelvic muscle to bring elasticity to the vaginal wall, which will increase sensation during sexual intercourse. Lie face down on the floor, arms to the side. Place your elbows under the shoulderblades with your palms face down and your fingers together. Inhale, push your palms and elbows down and lift your head up. Make sure your hip bones remain on the floor. Exhale and point your toes. ▸ Breathing normally, lift both legs up behind you, keeping your feet together. ▸ Balancing on your right arm, reach back with your left hand and take hold of your left foot. Lift your spine and look up. Hold for 5–7 seconds. Repeat on the other side.

3

BREAKS AND FRACTURES

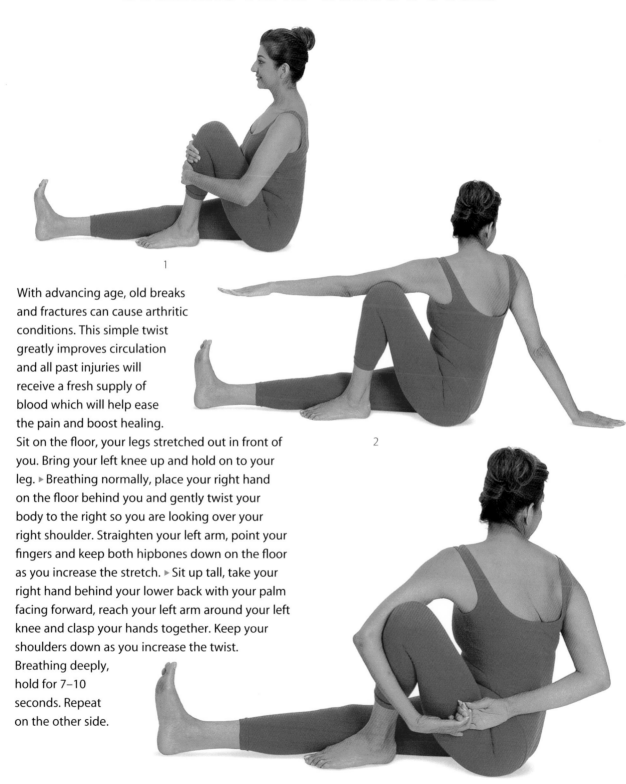

1

With advancing age, old breaks and fractures can cause arthritic conditions. This simple twist greatly improves circulation and all past injuries will receive a fresh supply of blood which will help ease the pain and boost healing.

Sit on the floor, your legs stretched out in front of you. Bring your left knee up and hold on to your leg. ▶ Breathing normally, place your right hand on the floor behind you and gently twist your body to the right so you are looking over your right shoulder. Straighten your left arm, point your fingers and keep both hipbones down on the floor as you increase the stretch. ▶ Sit up tall, take your right hand behind your lower back with your palm facing forward, reach your left arm around your left knee and clasp your hands together. Keep your shoulders down as you increase the twist. Breathing deeply, hold for 7–10 seconds. Repeat on the other side.

2

THYROID

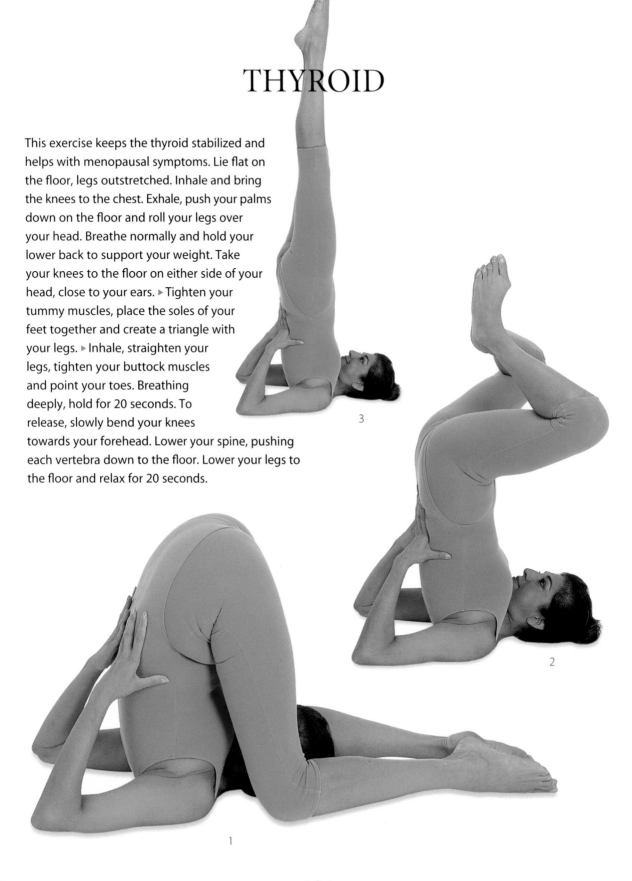

This exercise keeps the thyroid stabilized and helps with menopausal symptoms. Lie flat on the floor, legs outstretched. Inhale and bring the knees to the chest. Exhale, push your palms down on the floor and roll your legs over your head. Breathe normally and hold your lower back to support your weight. Take your knees to the floor on either side of your head, close to your ears. ▸ Tighten your tummy muscles, place the soles of your feet together and create a triangle with your legs. ▸ Inhale, straighten your legs, tighten your buttock muscles and point your toes. Breathing deeply, hold for 20 seconds. To release, slowly bend your knees towards your forehead. Lower your spine, pushing each vertebra down to the floor. Lower your legs to the floor and relax for 20 seconds.

3

2

1

DIGESTIVE

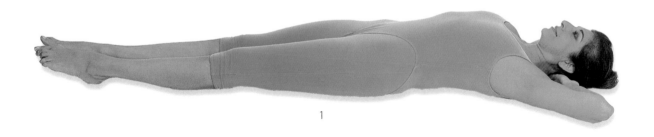

1

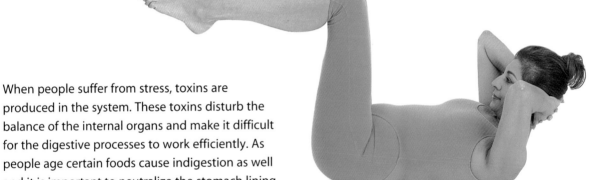

2

When people suffer from stress, toxins are produced in the system. These toxins disturb the balance of the internal organs and make it difficult for the digestive processes to work efficiently. As people age certain foods cause indigestion as well and it is important to neutralize the stomach lining and release gases from the bowel and digestive tract. This exercise will tone the whole digestive system. Lie flat on the floor. Point your toes and clasp your hands under your head. ▶ Inhale and simultaneously lift your head and legs up in a 90-degree angle. Exhale, breathe normally and hold for 5 seconds. ▶ Clasp your arms around your legs, holding on to your elbows. Tuck your forehead down to your knees. Point your toes and hold the position for 10 seconds. Slowly lower your spine to the floor and relax your legs down. Repeat the exercise and hold the position for 20 seconds, breathing deeply and evenly.

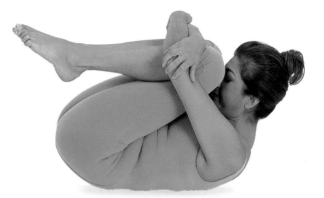

3

INDEX

ACKNOWLEDGEMENTS

Publishing Director

Laura Bamford

Commissioning Editor

Jane McIntosh

Editors

Catharine Davey

Diana Vowles

Creative Director

Keith Martin

Executive Art Editor

Mark Stevens

Designer

Louise Griffiths

Photography

Tim Ridley

Hair and Make-up

Bettina Graham

Production Controller

Julie Hadingham